The

Tao

of

Chi

Scott Shaw

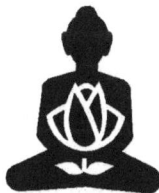

Buddha Rose Publications

First Edition 2013

ISBN: 1-877792-68-3
ISBN 13: 9781877792687
Library of Congress Control Number:
2013940473

Disclaimer: The practices, techniques, and
meditations presented in this book should not be used
as an alternative to professional medial treatment.
This book does not attempt to provide any medical
diagnosis treatments, prescriptions, or suggestions for
any medical issues of any kind. The techniques
presented in this book may be too strenuous for some
individuals. For this reason it is essential that you
consult your physician and receive his or her
permission before performing any of the techniques
detailed in this book. The author and the publishing
company are in no way responsible for any injury
you may cause yourself by practicing the techniques
presented in this book.

10 9 8 7 6 5 4 3 2 1

Printed in the United States of America

The Tao of Chi

Contents

Introduction

Modern science teaches us that every element of this universe, from the smallest subatomic particles to the largest planet, is pulsating with an energy. Over two thousand years ago, in ancient China, this energy was defined as Chi.

In the modern era, Chi is commonly understood to mean Internal Energy. Chi is much more than that, however. Chi is the universal energy that gives rise to all elements of life and fuels both the physical and spiritual universe.

Chi cannot be seen. Chi cannot be touched. Yet, those who have interacted with this universal energy can attest to the fact that it does, in fact, exist.

Because Chi is such an abstract science, many people believe that the ability to consciously access this energy is only available to monks who live in caves or advanced martial artists who practice esoteric styles of *Kung Fu*. This is not the case. The energy of Chi can be brought into the life of any individual who wished to perform a few simple exercises.

From the 3rd century B.C.E. forward, it has been understood that the human breath is what links the individual to the cosmic energy of Chi. From this knowledge, there have been very exacting techniques developed which instruct a person in how to effectively harness this power. These exercises are known by the Chinese term, *Chi Kung.*

The primary method to consciously bring the energy of Chi into the human body is via advanced methods of breath control. This science is based in the understanding that we, as human beings, are elementally dominated by breathing. We can live several days without food, a few without water, but the moment we are robbed of our breath, life, as we know it, ceases to exist.

With this imperative connection to breath as a basis of understanding, the ancient founders of *Chi Kung* acutely refined the methods for the intake of breath, whereby; the practitioner could come to a higher and more profound level of human interaction with the universal energy of Chi.

In the pages of this book, ancient method of *Chi Kung* will be detailed. From their practice, you will come to possess the ability to consciously become interactive with this universal energy and be able to tap into it in times of physical or mental need. By becoming consciously interactive with Chi you will be able to instantly summon up enhanced, and seemingly supernatural, amounts of physical and mental energy. No longer will you feel run down, lackadaisical, or spiritless. Instead, you will be filled with the vibrant source of energy which fuels this universe and you will be able to meet any challenge with dynamic physical power and positive mental focus.

1 Historical Foundations of Chi

The understanding of Chi was born in ancient China. This science came into existence with the indigenous Chinese religious philosophy of Taoism as its central determinate. The science of Chi, guided by Taoism and later Buddhism, has continually evolved throughout the centuries, directed not only by numerous teachers but various religious and social movements, as well. To help you to understand the process of evolution, which the science of Chi has undertaken, following are some of the motivating factors and ideologics embraced by the prominent schools and teachers of ancient times which were instrumental in moving this knowledge forward.

The Foundation of Chi
Though there is no exact date as to when the knowledge of Chi was initially embraced, the first text on the subject, *Huang Ti Nei Ching Su Wen, "The Yellow Emperor's Classic of Internal Medicine,"* was written during the Warring States period of Chinese history (401 - 223 B.C.E.).

Huang Ti Nei Ching Su Wen

In the *Huang Ti Nei Ching Su Wen,* Chi is described as the universal energy that nourishes and sustains all life. This text is written in the form of a dialogue on the subject of healing between, Huang-ti, the Yellow Emperor and his minister Chi-po.

Huang Ti

Huang-ti was a mythological ruler of China, legended to have lived from 2697 to 2599 B.C.E. He is said to have invented most aspects of Chinese culture. Though Chinese folklore claims this text was written during the mythical life of Huang-ti, its creation is historically dated at approximately 300 B.C.E.

Taoism

The primary philosophic system of belief present in China at the time when Chi understanding came to be embraced was that of Taoism. Taoism is a mystical school of thought that developed approximately five thousand years ago in the Chinese state of Ch'u, which is geographically located in the Yangtze Valley.

The Chinese term *Tao* refers to, *"Way." The Way* of existing in accordance with nature, internal and external harmony, and universal enlightened consciousness.

The understanding of Tao, through varying slightly from school to school, is a highly refined metaphysical method for the individual to leave behind the constrains of worldly consciousness and come into divine harmony with the universe. As Chi is the propelling factor of the universe, the followers of the Tao embraced this science and made the conscious interaction with Chi an integral part of their quest for divine interactive universal consciousness.

Lao Tsu

The ancient Sage Lao Tsu is credited with providing the first written definition for the understanding of Taoism, the *Tao Te Ching*. Though the date of his birth is unknown, his death is believed to have taken place in 604 B.C.E. The name Lao Tsu is translated from the Chinese as, *"Old Knower."*

Lao Tsu is believed to have been the custodian of the Royal Archives in the city of Loyang, the capital of the Chinese state of Ch'u. The primary legend about Lao Tsu states that he became despondent over the continued wars which were on-going during his lifetime and decided to renounce civilization and travel to the mountains to live his final days in meditative seclusion. As he was leaving the kingdom, a gatekeeper persuaded him to detail his wisdom for the benefit of mankind. This produced the most definitive work of Taoism, the *Tao Te Ching*.

The second prominent legend, propagated in China about Lao Tsu, is that once he imparted his knowledge to the gatekeeper he travelled on foot to India, where Siddhartha Guatama, the Sakyamuni Buddha became his student. To many believers of this legend this explains why the teachings of the Buddha so profoundly resemble those of mystical Taoism as they embraced the pursuit of cosmic nothingness.

Defining Lao Tsu

Lao Tsu is no doubt the most debated personage of Taoism. It would be unfair to not reveal the quandary over the facts of his existence. Some historians believe the *Tao Te Ching* was actually created in the third or fourth century B.C.E. by complying the works of several Taoist philosophers and was not the work of one single man. Whether this debate will ever be fully answered is yet to be determined. None-the-less the *Tao Te Ching* provided a philosophic basis for understanding that has elementally guided the development of all mystical schools of Chinese thought throughout history.

Tao Te Ching

The *Tao Te Ching* teaches a way existing in metaphysical non-action, known by the Chinese term, *"Wu Wei."* Within its pages it states that action removes one for the ultimate understanding of truth. For this reason, Taoist sages, throughout the centuries, have left behind worldly life and have journeyed deep into the wilderness in order to meditatively become one with the universe.

Kung Fu Tsu

Kung Fu Tsu, commonly known as Confucius by the English-speaking world, was the second personage to formally lay the foundations for Taoism. Kung Fu Tsu is believed to have been a younger contemporary of Lao Tsu – living from 551 to 479 B.C.E. Though Kung Fu Tsu's contribution was less dramatic to the overall growth of mystical Taoism, particular in relation to Chi, his teachings were, none-the-less, full of magical rites, many based in the understanding of Chi, which could be used to invoke and please Chinese Gods. In addition, his philosophy taught that high regard for the State and its royal leaders was elemental to an illuminated life. From feudal Chinese society onward, his writings, known as *Lun Yu, "Analects of Confucius,"* have been used to define Chinese statesmanship.

Chuang Tsu

Chuang Tsu (369-286 B.C.E.) was the third individual who's works substantially defined Taoism. Though born into a family of high standing, due to his refusal to serve any ruler, Chuang Tsu is believed to have lived modestly and worked as a minor administrative official in the city of Meng in the Honan Province of China.

Chuang Tsu's written work, *Nan Hua Chen Ching,* is commonly referred to in English as, *"The Inner Chapters."* The work metaphorically details how an individual should mindfully encounter the world. Chuang Tsu took up where Lao Tsu left off and detailed an exacting knowledge that, *"Universal Nothingness,"* known in Chinese by the word, *"Wu,"* must be embraced in order for one to come into contact with enlightened consciousness.

The Chinese term, *Chen Jen* or, *"Pure Human Being,"* was assigned to Chuang Tsu. This was due to the fact that he is understood to have become, *"One,"* with the Tao and embraced the illuminated knowledge of true spiritual freedom.

Meng Tsu

Meng Tsu (372 - 289 B.C.E.), more commonly known as Mencius, embraced and expounded upon the Confucian doctrines of Taoist understanding. Whereas, Chuang Tsu expanded the tenets of the mystical *Tao Te Ching* and embraced a highly metaphysical approach to life, the philosophy of Meng Tsu was rooted in his belief that man was inherently wise and good. His commentaries were based more in a reverence for Political State than of cosmic interactions, are left to that of philosophy. As such, he did little to expand the knowledge that each individual should focus his or her lives upon walking a refined path towards enlightenment based in interaction with Tao and Chi. None-the-less, he was historically a prominent teacher, leading to an ever evolving societal consciousness which expanded throughout ancient China.

Immortality

The primary goal of the early Taoist was to gain immortality. The Chinese term which describes this state of being is, *"Chang Sheng Pus Su."*

To the Taoist who focused their attention solely upon the spiritual understanding of this philosophy, immortality was exemplified by obtaining enlightenment. To the worldly Taoist, however, this pursuit was left to the realms of living forever in order to obtain extensive amounts of wealth and power. Whatever the motivation, the path to immortality became a highly defined science in ancient China, with the embracing of Chi as one of its primary components. It was firmly believed that if an individual could come upon the exact formula for the proper intake of herbs and minerals, in addition to performing exacting *Chi Kung* rituals, while living a life in accordance with the Tao, immortality could, in fact, be obtained.

Shen Hsien

The ancient Chinese text, *Shen Hsien,* was devoted entirely to the step-by-step method of how a human being could obtain immortality. Sadly, Emperor Chin Shih Huang-ti in the Third Century C.E destroyed this document, in association with numerous other ancient manuscripts. Thus, the world lost a great manuscript as to how the ancient Taoist viewed and practiced *Chi Kung.*

Wu Hsing

Wu Hsing, translated from the Chinese, literally means, *"Five Movers."* This term, however, is more commonly defined in Chinese understanding as, *"Five Virtues."* This being stated, in English, *Wu Hsing* would be better understood with the translation, *"Five Elements,"* as this concept details that five primary elements: water, fire, wood, metal, and earth which are believed to determine the course of human existence in this physical world.

These elements, which were historically understood to be the primary components of life, were more than simply aspects of this physical world. They were, in fact, perceived as metaphysical components that defined the course of humanity.

The Five Elements are a complex understanding of movement and interrelationships. Each element has the potential to give birth to or destroy another. Wood gives birth to fire, fire to earth, earth to metal, and metal to water. Water annihilated fire, fire overcame metal, metal overpowered wood, wood vanquishes earth, and earth destroys water.

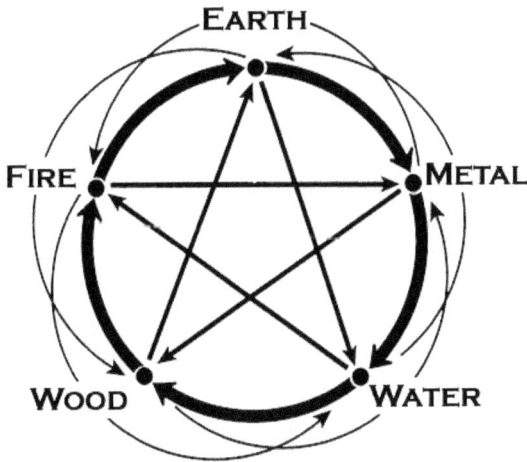

These *Five Elements* were additionally defined as possessing a color, direction, and texture. Fire embodied the color red, pointed South, and emanated a bitter taste. Earth was the Northern direction, black in color, and possessed the taste of salt. Wood was East, the color green, and held a sour taste. Metal shown

West, was white in color, and had a powerful taste. And finally, water was directed towards the center of the universe, yellow in color, and had a sweet taste.

Each of these *Five Elements* was also responsible for a specific function of the human body. If an individual became sick it was understood that they were out of alignment with a specific element. The element of fire was responsible for the heart, the small intestines, and the blood vessels. Water took care of the skeletal structure, the kidneys, the bladder, and the ears. Earth oversaw the stomach, the pancreas, the muscles of the body, and the mouth. Wood was in charge of the gall bladder, the liver, and the eyes. Metal dominated of the large intestines, the lungs, and nose.

The Five Elements also had specific emotion linked to them: joy was related to fire, sadness to metal, fear to water, worrying to earth, and anger to wood.

To the modern individual this style of defining human existence by assigning aspects, believed to be inherent to these *Five Elements* may seem strange. From a scientific perspective this may be a correct assumption. It must be understood, however, that more than simply the superficial aspects of fire, water, wood, earth, and metal, these *Five Elements* were seen as possessing intimate metaphysical qualities. For this reason, the people of that ancient time period used them as a way of defining the unknown and the yet undiscovered aspects of their lives. Thus, these *Five Elements* were a means of placing meaning into a world dominated by a lack of scientific understanding.

Tsou Yen

Tsou Yen (350 - 270 B.C.E) is oftentimes credited as the inventor of *The Five Element* understanding. Tsou Yen applied this teaching to all things known to man. He classified Chinese history, geography, people, animals, and vegetables, assigning each a specific component of the five elements.

Wu Tao Mi Tao

The ancient Sage, Chang Tao Ling (34 - 156 C.E.) was one of the first proponents of the Common Era to move the understanding of Chi to new levels of acceptance. He was the founder of, *Wu Tao Mi Tao*, literally *"Five Pecks of Rice Taoism,"* This sect is more commonly known as, *"School of the Celestial Masters."* It remained in existence until the Fifteenth Century.

Chang Tao Ling embraced the teaching of *Tao Te Ching* and was a healer by trade. He believed, as did many of his time, that illness was caused by evil deeds. Chi Tao Ling cured people by performing magical incantations over them, providing them with talismans, and holy water. Each of these remedies was understood to transcend their common physical components and be, in fact, manifestations of positive Chi energy.

The charge for his services; five pecks of rice. Thus, the name of the school.

Yu Chi

Yu Chi (124 - 197 C.E.) was another early Common Era Master of *Chi Kung* whose teachings laid the foundation for later schools of Taoist Chi evolution. Legend states that Yu Chi came into possession of the definitive text, *Tai Ping Ching Ling Shu, "Book of Supreme Peace and Purity,"* via a miracle, in approximately 145 C.E. This book became the primary doctrine for many later schools of mystical Taoism.

Yu Chi spent his life as a healer, curing people through Chi manipulation, holy water purification, and herbs. Ironically, a family member at the height of his national popularity killed him.

Tai Ping Tao

During the Second Century C.E., Chang Chueh (114-184 C.E.) founded, *Tai Ping Tao, "The Way of Supreme Peace"* school of Taoism. He based his philosophy on a combination of the *Huang Ti Nei Ching Su Wen* and a loose interpretation of the *Tao*

Te Ching. The primary doctrine for the school was Yu Chi's, *Tai Ping Ching Ling Shu, "Book of Supreme Peace and Purity."* The influence of Chang Chueh spread across eight political districts of China, making his school one of the most important religious sects of this time period.

Tai Ping Tao initially came to be embraced by the masses due to the abilities of Chang Chueh as a healer. It was his belief that the first step for the ill person to become well was for them to confess their sins. This was due to the fact that the mental anguish caused by sins set Chi out of balance that was the root of all illness. Once confession was publicly performed, Chang Chueh could then effectively heal the individual through a combination of *Chai "Fasting," Fu Lu "Talismans," Fu Shui "Holy water,"* and Chi manipulation based upon *Huang Ti Nei Ching Su Wen.*

During the lifetime of Chang Chueh, China was not only plagued by disease and famine but the heartless rule of the corrupt Han Dynasty (202 B.C.E - 220 C.E.), as well. Based in no small part on the socioeconomic conditions which surrounded him, Chang Chueh, taught a method of spirituality whereby his devotees could enter into a meditative state and be released from the pains of the physical world.

Chang Chueh was a formidable figure in the foundations of spiritual Taoism, he was also much more than a simple religious teacher – he was a political activist, as well. Chang Chueh formed the pro-active political group known as the Yellow Turbans, *"Huang Chin"* and proclaimed himself the Celestial Duke General. With the guidance of Chang Chueh, the Yellow Turbans set about to overthrow the Han Dynasty. It was the belief of Chang Chueh that in the year 184 the Han Dynasty could be toppled, thereby giving birth to an age of supreme peace. To this end, Chang Chueh organized his followers into a Chinese hierarchical force, with himself and his two brothers: Chang Pao, the Terrestrial Duke General and Chang Liang, the People's Duke General, as the leaders. In 184 Chang Chueh lead the Huang Chin rebellion against the Han. The Yellow Turbans were ruthlessly defeated, however, and Chang Chueh, his brothers, and most of his disciples were killed.

Chang Liang

One of Chang Chueh's primary foes was Chang Liang (100 - 187 C.E.). Chang Liang was a high-level government minister in the Han Cabinet who was deeply rooted in the Kung Fu Tsu ideology of Taoism that proclaimed that divine respect should be afforded to all governmental officials. He sought to destroy any teaching to the commoners, such as those of Chang

Chueh's, which were not directly linked to the Confucian Taoism propagated by the Han Dynasty, as he believed that commoners were too lowly to truly understand Taoism and, thus, should only be allowed to worship those of royal heritage. In an interesting twist of historic fate, Chinese history would proclaim Chang Liang to be one of the first individuals to obtain spiritual immortality due to his practice of *Tiao Yin, (detailed in Chapter 3),* and give him the title, *Tao Chiao, "Founder of Religious Taoism."*

Cheng-i Tao

Ching-i Tao or *"Way of Right Union,"* was an important sect of Taoism founded during the Second Century C.E.

This school employed talismans, amulets, and precisely drawn magical symbols in order to not only activate Chi but to bring an individual into closer union with divine consciousness.

This sect is considered as a form of religious Taoism and was highly embraced by the superstitious masses of the time period. The practices of *Cheng-i Tao* have been embraced up to the modern era and have come to define much of the Chinese mindset in relation to use of external objects in order to gain favour from the Gods and deities.

Yin Yang Chia

During the Third Century C.E. *Yin Yang Chia, "Yin and Yang Sect"* came into prominence as a central focus of philosophic understanding among the Taoist elite. This school adopted the ancient Chinese philosophic concept of Yin and Yang and taught that the universe arose from the interplay of these two energies, both on the physical and spiritual level.

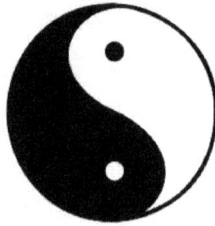

Yin and Yang, literally translated from Chinese means, *"Shade and light."* In its most ancient format, *Yin and Yang* was used to define the fact of whether or not there was sunlight on the fertile mountain slopes where agricultural farming took place. *Yang* was used to denote the mountain slope that faced the sun and *Yin* to define the slope of the mountain facing away from the sun. As time progressed in ancient China, the concept of Yin and Yang took on a much more philosophic understanding of defining the polarizing elements of the universe: White and Black, Positive and Negative, Light and Heavy, Female and Male, Heaven and Earth.

The first written document detailing *Yin and Yang* occurred in the oracle Chinese text, *I Ching, "Book of Changes,"* created in approximately 1100 B.C.E., during the transition between the Yin and the Chou dynasties. The *I Ching* was one of the few Chinese texts to survive the burning of all ancient manuscripts, ordered by the first historical emperor of China, Chin Shih Huang-ti in 213 C.E.

As the Han Dynasty (202 B.C.E. - 220 C.E.) came to prominence and the Chinese Empire rose to it pinnacle, *Yin Yang Chia* began to incorporate the understanding of *Wu Hsing "Five Elements,"* into its overall teachings.

Chu Lin Chi Hsien

Whereas, the school of *Yin Yang Chia,* during the third century, embraced a relatively sedate philosophic approach to metaphysical involvement with Chi and nature, *Chu Lin Chi Hsien* or *"Seven Sages of the Bamboo Grove,"* took on a much more radical approach. This group of Taoist holy men not only were talented musicians and artists but they believed by the excessive consumption of wine, they could ultimately become one with the universe.

Huang Ting Ching

The third century C.E. was a period which witnessed vast expansion in the philosophic understanding of the individual in association with Chi. *Huang Ting Ching* or "Treatise on the Yellow Hall" is a text, written during this period, which describes *Chi Kung* understanding whereby the individual will reach immortality.

This text's primary focus was teaching that the breath, as understood to be the primary component of bringing Chi into the human being, must be allowed to flow unhindered through the entire body, as detailed in *Chi Kung* exercises such as *Lien Chi* (see Chapter 11). From this, the practitioner would not only have superhuman energy, but also would regain youth, and eventually become immortal.

Hsuan Hsueh

Another school active during the third, and into the forth, century was *Hsuan Hseuh,* which literally means, *"Secret Mystical Teachings."* This sect of mystical Taoists combined the teachings of Lao Tsu and Chuang Tsu and blended them with the principals of Kung Fu Tsu's worship of higher deities. This group, due to their blending of philosophies, became known as a Neo-Taoist movement.

One of their primary proponents of this sect was Wang Ti (226 - 249 C.E.). He was instrumental in creating *Ching Tan* or *"Pure Conversation."* This was a highly refined method of articulation whereby members of this group could communicate on the tenets of Taoism in an acutely refined manner.

Throughout history, the mystical Taoists believed that Lao Tsu was the highest of all Sages who walked upon the Earth. Wang Ti, on the other hand, taught that Kung Fu Tsu was, in fact, a higher being and that he was the one who had obtained *Wu, "Cosmic Nothingness."* *Wu* being the most sought after metaphysical state.

Due to the ever evolving metaphysical consciousness in China at this time, teachings provided by schools such as *Hsuan Hseuh* began to place more and more focus upon actively seeking *Wu* and the *"Spiritual Emptiness"* provided by meditation. From this, Buddhism began to be embraced by these Neo-Taoist schools and later came to be commonly integrated with many sects of Taoism.

Buddhism

Buddhism was born in India. Siddhartha Guatama (563-483 B.C.E.), a prince from the Northern region of the India Subcontinent, left behind his royal lifestyle to become a *Sadhu, "A wandering practitioner of Yoga."* Upon reaching enlightenment and becoming a spiritual teacher, he lay the foundation for the religion which was later to be formulated around his teachings.

As mentioned, legend states that the Chinese Sage Lao Tsu may have, in fact, been a teacher of Siddhartha Guatama, known as the Sakyamuni Buddha, *"The enlightened one from the clan of Sakya."* This lore, however, will probably never be historically proven. None-the-less, due to the similarities possessed between Taoism and Buddhism – the quest of the human being entering into a state of divine nothingness and becoming one with the cosmic whole, Buddhism was embraced in China, with varying degrees of success, from the first century of the Common Era onwards. During the third century, however, Buddhism firmly took hold in China, and found futile ground for its evolution.

Buddhabhadra

One of the early Buddhist zealots to journey from India to China and embrace the science of breath control used for the enhancement of Chi into the human body was Buddhabhadra (359-429). Though select Buddhist monks had commonly travelled to China in the early centuries of the Common Era to propagate the understanding of Buddhism, most spent their days lost deeply in meditation and working at the task of translating the Buddhist Scriptures into Chinese. The majority of these early monks were not practitioners of either the ancient *yogic* methods of breath control, known as *Pranayama* or Chinese *Chi Kung*. Buddhabhadra was the exception to this rule.

Buddhabhadra was of the Hinayana sect of Buddhism and he practiced a style of meditation known as *Dharmatrata Dhyana*. This method of meditation possessed a primary component of breath control. From his refined practices he came to be known, throughout China, as possessing supernatural powers. Thus, he helped to lay the foundation for the science of Chi to be embraced by Buddhist practitioner, as well as Taoists.

Ta Moo

The legendary Buddhist monk, Ta Moo, (more commonly known as Bodhidharma), was born in Kanchipuram, India, near modern day Madras. He renounced the princely status he possessed in order to follow the path of Tantric Buddhism – which embraced the understanding that enlightenment came to the zealot via an instantaneous experience of realization.

In 520 C.E. Ta Moo was sent to China by his Guru, Prajnatara to relieve the Indian Buddhist monk, Bodhiruci and become the Abbott of the *Shongshan Monastery,* (also referred to as the Shaolin Temple in the modern era). As Ta Moo belonged to the *Sarvastivada Sect* of

Buddhism, which practiced an approach to Buddhism with the embracing of consciousness nothingness at its source, the Chinese readily accepted Ta Moo's teachings as they closely parallel the mystical understanding inherent to Taoism.

Upon arrival at the monastery, Ta Moo found that the monastic life had left the Chinese monks weak and in ill health. To remedy their physical condition he taught them a series of breath control exercises based in the yogic understanding of *pranayama,* which is similar in many ways to the Chinese understanding of *Chi Kung.* The two primary exercises he is credited with developing are *Yin Jin Jing, "Muscle and Tendon Changing"* and *Hsi Sui Jing, "Marrow and Brain Cleansing."* Many *Chi Kung* exercises have evolved from these two ancient techniques, particularly the *Chi Kung* exercise, known as *Tao Yin,* which is detailed in *Chapter 5.*

The Shaolin Temple

In the modern era much has been written and depicted about the now infamous *Shongshan (Shaolin) Temple.* Many would-be historians have dated the inception of the various martial art systems, collectively known as *Kung Fu,* (more correctly *Wu Shu),* to the initial teachings of Ta Moo at this monastery. Historically, however, various forms of the martial arts were widely practiced throughout Asia long before the time of Ta Moo.

Emperor Hsiao Wen commissioned *The Shaolin Temple* in the late fifth century. Its name is derived from the surrounding forest of tress that crept up to the walls of the monastery. It was located in the Honan Province, Tung Feng region, of China. It was constructed to honor the contributions made by Ta Moo's predecessor, Bodhiruci.

As the centuries progressed, the Buddhist teaching which Bodhiruci and Ta Moo propagated at the *Shaolin Temple* spread out across China. Numerous sects sprung from these mystical understandings. Some of the followers who were directly linked to these teachings held onto the temple's name and constructed new branches in various geographic locations throughout China. This was a source of the continued evolution of Chi knowledge.

As China moved forward into the modern era, the *Shaolin Temple* became a politically orientated institution, especially during its later years. During this time it was primarily used as a training ground for anti-governmental revolutionaries, just prior to, and during the *Boxer Revolution* (1898-1900). *The Boxer Revolution* witnessed all foreign missionaries and business people driven out of China.

Though the *Shaolin Temple* was certainly not the only source of *Chi Kung* and Martial Art evolution in China, it has remained a romanticized central focal point due to media interpretations.

Tao Hong Jing

Tao Hong Jing (462-547 C.E.) was a famed healer, advanced herbalist, and an influential Chi Kung master who influenced the further development of the understanding. He wrote several books that came to define the mastery of Chi during this period of time and helped to evolve the science for centuries to come. Among his works was, *Yang Shen Tao Ying Tu, "The Manual of Heath Preserving Breathing Exercises."*

Tao Hong Jing taught that for one to maintain optimum health and posses a constant interaction with Chi, they must meditate daily and focus their attention on Chi entering the body through the breath. He also taught that one should practice sexual abstinence. From this, the vital energy of the body would remain intact, causing Chi to circulate more fervently.

Tao Hong Jin believed that for one to maintain optimum health and maximum Chin interaction they must stand with a straight posture and walk with a consciousness of nature and Chi. If one were to become ill, he instructed them to meditate, focus Chi on the location of their ailment and consciously breathe Chi to this location.

Zhi Yu

As detailed, Buddhism played an important role in the evolution of *Chi Kung* throughout China. The Buddhist monk Zhi Yu lived during the early stages of *The Five Dynasty Period* (581-979 C.E.). He was very influential in expanding the understanding of the interrelationship between meditation and *Chi Kung*. He devised an exercise known as *Zhi Chaun Fa*. *Zhi Chaun Fa* which lead the practitioner into a deep state of meditation by having them focus their attention upon their breath. It was designed to then systematically free the practitioner from desire by focusing Chi on the six physical canters of desire.

These bodily locations are more commonly known as the chakras. There are normally seven chakras detailed. Zhi Yu did not recognize the seventh chakra located on the crown of the head, however, as no desire is held in this energy center for this is the bodily location where cosmic consciousness may be encountered.

By first obtaining a deep state of meditation and then focusing Chi on the center of desire, Zhi Yu taught that desire was literally burned out of the practitioner through the positive power of Chi.

Zim Chueng Shen

Zim Chueng Shen was a *Chi Kung* master who lived during the early part of the Tang Dynasty (618 - 906 C.E.). He taught that the eating of meat was adverse to not only a person's health but to their conscious interaction with Chi, as well. He based his premise on that fact that all elements of this universe, both animate and inanimate, are alive and thriving with Chi. If you take the life of an animal and cause his Chi to stop flowing, then you have altered the natural balance of the universe. If you then go on to eat the animal, you are consuming a very negative from of Chi which will not only effect your later interaction with Chi but will cause you to become prone to illness due to ingesting a substance with non-active Chi.

Zim Chueng Shen taught that there were five steps to obtain conscious Chi interaction.

1. Observe your body as sacred vessel. Do not eat meat and drink wine.

2. Find a solitary place and practice Chi Kung daily.

3. Meditate. Stop thinking, seeking new experiences, and storing thoughts, for they will cause you nothing but grief.

4. Sit and Forget. Forget both you and me. Forget heaven and earth. Forget all things.

5. All things can be known if you touch the source of Chi. You can control Yin and Yang and exist in the every-lasting universe.

Zim Chueng Shen wrote many texts on Chi Kung and meditation. Perhaps his most profound work was entitled, *Zhou Wang Lun, "Sitting and Forgetting."*

Lung Dong Bin
Lung Dong Bin was one of the most influential teachers of Chi Kung during the early Tang Dynasty. He wrote, *Bai Zui Bei, "The One-hundred Word Epitaph."* In this one-hundred word manuscript he poetically states that one should refrain from doing anything that is not absolutely necessary and that every movement should possess a reason. And that, all you should do with your life is stop speaking, meditate, and encounter Chi.

Wu Tsung
Emperor Wu Tsung (814 - 850 C.E.) was one of the key foes against the proliferation of Buddhism throughout China. He was an Emperor of the Tang Dynasty. During the reign of this dynasty, the China Empire was the largest and wealthiest on

earth. Arts and philosophy flourished and the knowledge of Chi was highly embraced.

Wu Tsung was a staunch supporter of Taoism. As such, he saw to it that many of the Buddhist temples located in China were destroyed and many of its adherents put to death. Thus, demonstrating how the philosophic inclinations of a political leader could truly affect the evolution of religion. From the acts of Wu Tsung, many of the Buddhist orientated Chi development understandings were left to monks who went into hiding in caves in the mountains and practiced their techniques in secret.

Yun Chi – Chi Chien

Yun Chi – Chi Chien, "The Cloud Book and Seven Strips of Bamboo," is one of the most important canons composed on the subject of *Chi Kung*. Written in the eleventh century, this text details all of the known exercises of Taoist *Chi Kung* through the Song Dynasty (960 - 1279). In addition, it details biographies and medical practices common to the Chinese foundations of Chi.

Tai-i Tao

Hsiao Pao Chen was the founder of the *Tai-i Tao, "Way of the Supreme Tao"* school of Taoism. Though the school was a sect of metaphysical Taoism, it possessed much reverence for the works of Kung Fu

Tsu. Thus, it bridged the gap between religious and political Taoism.

Hsiao Pao Chen found much of his inspiration from the *Cheng-i Tao, "Way of Just Unity"* school of Taoism. Thus, Hsiano's disciples were active participant of *Fu Lu Pai, "Magical or Alchemistic Taoism."*

The primary deity this school worshiped was, *Huang Lao Chun, "Ancient Yellow Lord,"* who was believed to have descended to earth several times in order to help mankind. Lao Tsu was believed to be one of his incarnations.

Tai-i Tao was a strictly monastic sect of Taoism. Its followers believed that one could not achieve the higher realms of consciousness or immortality if they were burdened by the demands of society. Thus, they retreated to monasteries to heighten their meditative and Chi awareness and hone their alchemistic skills. The sect fell into decline during the Yuan Dynasty (1279 - 1368 C.E.).

Tai-i Chin Hua Tsung Chih

Tai-i Chin Hua Tsung Chih or *"The Golden Flower of the Supreme One,"* is a Seventeenth Century text detailing highly exacting techniques of *Chi Kung* and meditation. It teaches that the inner light of Chi can be trained to consciously circulate in your body thus creating the *"Golden*

Flower;" a symbolic term detailing your pure inner spirit merging with the cosmic whole, creating a divine union.

Chi in the Modern Era

As the centuries progressed, the science of Chi was passed on and advanced not only within China, but in Korea and Japan, as well. The techniques of *Chi Kung,* once believed only masterable by monks and holy men, have evolved to the state where today, this ancient knowledge can be accessed by anyone who takes the time to consciously come into an interactive relationship with this universal energy.

2 Chi Kung Preparation

Chi is science that has been practiced and handed down for centuries. Similar to the music that comes from the speakers of your stereo, Chi cannot be seen but can be experienced. As Chi cannot be physically seen or touched, by the untrained individual, there are many who do not believe in the power of this ancient understanding.

Chi is a mental science. As such, to begin to experience its power, you must initially possess at least a general belief in this understanding. From this step of faith, once you begin the practices of *Chi Kung,* detailed in this book, you will quickly begin to encounter the power of this ancient knowledge.

Preparing to Touch Chi

Though Chi is universally available, most people do not understand how to readily access this energy. Therefore, throughout the centuries there have been exacting methods devised which bring you into contact with this energy in the most expedient fashion possible.

To begin your practice of *Chi Kung* there are a few preliminary understandings you must possess. By employing these techniques you will begin to come into conscious contact with Chi. Thus, you will bypass many of the obstacles that have the potential to keep you from rapidly becoming empowered with this universal energy.

Chi and Your Breath

You can live a few days without water, several without food, but you can only exist for a few moments without air. The air you breathe is the most vital key to your life.

You can expand upon this basis of knowledge by looking to modern medical science and viewing the statistics that the individual who is actively involved in cardio vascular activities is the least prone to many types of physical and mental ailments. Thus, from a strictly scientific point of view, those who take in the most oxygen are the healthiest.

With this as a basis of understanding, the *Chi Kung* practitioner actively brings in excess amounts of oxygen into their body. They do not do this from solely an athletic vantage point, but instead from very refined methods of breath control. Thus, the ancient science of *Chi Kung* teaches what modern medicine has, only in the recent past; begin to understand – oxygen is good.

Chi Kung teaches that Chi is consciously brought into your body via your breath. The *Chi Kung* practitioner comes to understand that no longer is breathing simply an unconscious act. Instead, it is embraced as a pathway to not only enhanced physical and mental well being but also a way to come into contact with the divine energy of this universe, as well.

The Two Breaths of Chi

There are two distinct techniques of breathing directly associated with *Chi Kung*. The first is *Zhen Hu Zi, "Normal Breathing"* and the second is *Fan Hu Zi, "Reverse Breathing."*

Normal breathing is the natural pattern of breathing. When you breathe in, your chest and stomach expand. This style of breathing, when used in association with *Chi Kung,* is also known as, *"Buddha Breathing,"* as this was the style of breathing used by ancient Buddhist practitioners of *Chi Kung.*

Reverse Breathing is the process of reversing this natural process – when a breath comes in, your chest and stomach contract. This style of breathing, also known as *"Taoist Breathing,"* as this was the style of breath the ancient Taoist practitioners of *Chi Kung* put to use.

Proponents of each style of *Chi Kung Breathing* will argue their case as to the superiority of their method over the other. If we look at nature, however, we see that a baby's chest naturally expands when they breathe in. With this as our guide, it is suggested that you breathe in the natural pattern when practicing the *Chi Kung* techniques presented in this book. As it is believed that you should allow the natural process inherent to nature to ultimately be your guide in relation to Internal Energy.

The Two Types of Chi

There are two distinct types of Chi that are linked to the practices of *Chi Kung*. The first is known as, *Wai Chi* or *"Outer Chi,"* and the second is *Nei Chi* or *"Internal Chi."*

Wai Chi is the Chi that empowers the universe around you. This is the Chi that you consciously take in through your breath when you perform *Chi Kung. Wai Chi* is the element of Chi that provides you with a new and unlimited source of energy.

Nei Chi or Internal Chi is the energy that you consciously unleash into your body, from your central energy point. The techniques associated with this process will be discussed in the pages that follow.

Two Types of Chi Kung

There are two specific styles of *Chi Kung*. They are, *Tung Kung, "Active,"* and *Ching Kung, "Passive."*

Active *Chi Kung* represents the methods of breath control from either standing, seated, or lying positioning. These are the exercises that directly cause Chi to rapidly come into and effectively circulate throughout your body.

The practitioner who, through years of practice, has transcended the need for additional amounts of Chi to nourish their internal or external beings, on the other hand, utilizes passive Chi Kung. This occurs when you have purified your body to the degree that Chi has permeated your being. Thus, you are constantly interactive and, in fact, a direct channel for this cosmic energy. At this point, your only focus is upon that of meditation.

Sitting

When you perform seated *Chi Kung,* it is advisable that you sit in the cross-legged *Lotus Posture.* The reason for this is that this posture naturally *"Locks"* Chi energy into your upper torso. As several Meridians end in your legs or feet, Chi energy, which has been consciously brought into your body, has the potential to escape unnoticed via these bodily elements.

As seated *Chi Kung* techniques were designed to be practiced in this fashion for highly refined reasons, unnatural loss of Chi will cause your *Chi Kung* exercise to provide less than adequate results. The *Lotus Posture* naturally keeps this form occurring.

Many people, due to age, arthritis, or previous injuries have trouble sitting in this positioning. If this is your case, there are two things you can do. One, slowly develop the ability to sit in this posture by short periods of practice. When you are doing this, you will not want to attempt to perform *Chi Kung* because the discomfort you are experiencing will distract you from the actual technique and your results will be substantially minimized. Simply sit and attempt to become comfortable with this posture.

The second thing you can do is to sit in a chair with your spine erect. The best way to keep your body consciousness at its pinnacle, while performing *Chi Kung* from this positioning, is to sit several inches away from the back of the chair. From sitting in this fashion, you will not become relaxed.

If you perform seated *Chi Kung* in this manner, you must remain very conscious about the possibility of escaping Chi particularly via your feet. Therefore, it is important to wrap a blanket or towel around your feet if your practice seated *Chi Kung* in this manner. This should be done no matter what temperature it is outside.

The reason this is put into effect is that with your feet naturally warmed, Chi energy will not naturally flow to that region of your body attempting to warm it. Thus, you will be saved from unnecessary Chi loss.

Standing

Many *Chi Kung* exercises are performed from a stationary standing positioning. As all *Chi Kung* practices are performed with interactive mental consciousness as the elementary focus. This is also the case with *Chi Kung* standing. When you stand to perform *Chi Kung,* it is not simply standing in the ordinary sense – you must stand very consciously.

When you enter into your standing positioning, do not just stand – enter into this posture as if you are standing for the first time. Move into the positioning experiencing every element of your physical being. How do your feet, ankles, legs, and hips feel? As *Chi Kung* is an advanced level of human interaction with universal energy, truly knowing your body is the first step in entering into mutual relationship.

The physical posture of *Chi Kung* standing witnesses your spine straight but not unnaturally forced into an erect positioning. Your legs are naturally separated at approximately shoulder level. Your knees are never locked but allowed to have a very gentle bend. Your arms are placed freely to your sides, your fingers loosely extended. Your gaze should be naturally forward, never unduly focused on any specific physical object.

Your Tongue, Teeth, and Eyes

When you perform *Chi Kung* exercises your tongue should be lightly placed against the top of your mouth. This causes the *Yin and Yang,* polarizing energies of your body, to meet and intermingle in a harmonious fashion.

Your teeth should be allowed to lightly touch in a natural pattern.

Generally during *Chi Kung* your eyes will be closed in a natural fashion. At the outset of many of the exercises, however, your eyes will be open as you begin to take control and focus your mental energy. In these time periods, as limited as they may be, it is important not to visually focus upon any specific physical object. As everything in this universe is composed of an energy, you do not wish to take undue amounts of any undefined energy into your being prior to your *Chi Kung* practices. Thus, allow your eyes to randomly focus as your attention draws inward.

The Meridians

Chi permeates every aspect of every element of this universe. As such, Chi is present in every molecule of your human body. Though it is universally present in your being, it travels along exacting pathways known in Chinese as *Jing.*

Jing, or as they are commonly referred to in English, *"Meridians"* are invisible channels inside your body. They function in much the same way as does your blood vessels. Whereas blood circulates throughout your entire body via your blood vessels, Chi travels via your Meridians.

Each organ of the human body has a Meridian that governs the flow of Chi to and from it. When you are in balance, your Meridian channels are open and Chi nourishes your organs and the various body functions they each individually effect. When you are out of balance your body shows symptoms of physical and emotional illness, which indicates one or more of your Meridians has become blocked.

The Constant Meridians

There are a total of twelve *Constant Meridians* which function within each human body. These twelve are referred to as *Constant Meridians* because Chi energy circulates through them in a constant and continual delineated path. Of these twelve; ten are defined by the specific organ of the human body that they dominate.

They are:
Dan Jing,
    "Gall Bladder Meridian,"

Gan Jing,
> *"Liver Meridian,"*

Fei Jing,
> *"Lung Meridian,"*

Da Chang Jing,
> *"Large Intestine Meridian,"*

Xian Chang Jing,
> *"Small Intestine Meridian,"*

Wei Jing,
> *"Stomach Meridian,"*

Pi Jing,
> *"Spleen Meridian,"*

Xin Jing,
> *"Heart Meridian,"*

Pang Guang Jing,
> *"Bladder Meridian,"*

Shun Jing,
> *"Kidney Meridian."*

The final two *Constant Meridians: Xin Bao Jing, "Heart Constrictor Meridian,"* which regulates the sexual and reproductive Chi energy in a person and, *Sao Jian Jing, "Triple Warmer Meridian,"* which dominates three specific functions of the body: the energy of respiration, the control of digestion, and the control of body discharges, are related to the control of bodily functions.

Each of these *Constant Meridians* possesses a location on both the right side and the left side of your body. Through the practices of *Chi Kung,* your Meridians are stimulated and thus remain balanced and open with a constant flow of Chi traveling through them.

The Secondary Meridians

There are two additional Meridians that also aid in the control and circulation of Chi throughout your body. These *Secondary Meridians* influence highly specific Chi channels and bodily activities. Thus, they are referred to as *"Secondary Meridians."* They are the *Conceptual Meridian,* which is responsible for balancing the overall functioning of your body, and the Governing *Vessel Meridian,* which nourishes and aligns the other Meridians.

Chi and Your Environment

The benefits you will gain from *Chi Kung* are directly related to the physical environment where you practice, the type of food that you eat, and the type of lifestyle you live. If you are in a noisy, dirty, or polluted environment, eating bad food, drinking bad drink, and associating with negative people, your mind will not only be unduly distracted but your physical body will be suffering due to the impure surrounding you have placed yourself in.

It is essential to know, as you begin on your path to Chi consciousness that you are in control of your life. Therefore, you can focus your energy and move your

physical being to any place you desire.
Allow the *Chi Kung* techniques in this book
to help you focus your life and move you to
a placement and position where all the
positive energy of the universe can
embellish you.

The Energy Meridians

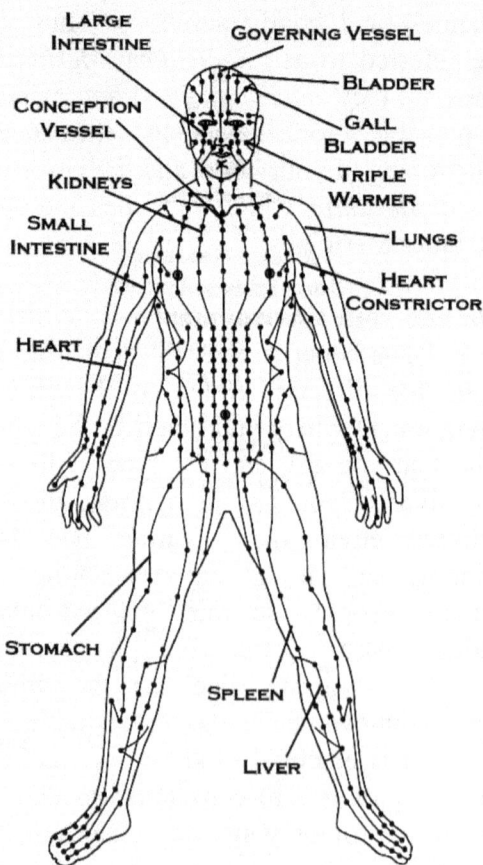

LARGE INTESTINE
GOVERNNG VESSEL
BLADDER
CONCEPTION VESSEL
GALL BLADDER
KIDNEYS
TRIPLE WARMER
SMALL INTESTINE
LUNGS
HEART CONSTRICTOR
HEART
STOMACH
SPLEEN
LIVER

Chi and Personal Power

Chi Kung is a process of body and mind purification and enhancement, not a method to direct excess amounts of Chi into your body so that you can physically or mentally overpower others. Do not practice it with the hopes of gaining some mythical power in order to dominate others or your practice will be fruitless.

There is a natural balance in this universe. If any person attempts to gain or maintain control over another, this balance is set out of alignment and the power-seeking individual quickly falls from their superior positioning. For this reason, the pure *Chi Kung* practitioner only practices the exercises as a means of coming into a more conscious interaction with the positive energies of this universe. From this, they can help all of humanity move to a more conscious plane of divine interaction.

3 Tiao Chi

Tiao Chi is translated from Chinese as, *"The Harmonizing of the Breath."*

Breath is what brings Chi into your body. When you refine your breathing techniques to an exacting science, enhanced amounts of Chi can be consciously taken into your being to aid you in times of physical or mental need.

The *Tiao Chi* exercise is the first or preliminary breathing technique that you must become familiar with before attempting to perform any further forms of *Chi Kung.* From this exercise, your breath and your body are brought into conscious harmony and universal Chi may enter and travel through your being unhindered.

Chi Blockage

The reason that it is necessary to perform this exercise before proceeding further with *Chi Kung,* is that if there is any hindrance to the flow of Chi along any Meridian channel in your body, the enhanced intake of Chi may reach an impasse point and cause a Chi build up in that specific bodily region. This can have an injurious effect to the overall Chi flow throughout your entire being.

The causation factors which have the potential to develop a Chi blockage are: the long term intake of improper food or drink, breathing polluted air over an extended period of time, an unhealed injury to a specific bodily part, or a unexercised aging body. If a Chi blockage has occurred, it means that you are out of balance with nature. Thus, if you perform *Chi Kung* before your body is freed from this blockage, the potential is substantially heightened that you will be thrown further out of balance with the specific Yin or Yang energy common to your obstructed Meridian and freeing that blockage will become increasingly complicated.

For this reason, *Tiao Chi* is always performed prior to any, more advanced, *Chi Kung* practices in order to open your Meridian pathways and allow Chi to enter and successfully flow throughout your being, unhindered.

Due to the very subtle effective nature of this technique it is often times referred to as, *Tong Guan* or *"Opening the Gate."*

Tiao Chi: Exercise One

To begin the *Tiao Chi* exercise, stand up and loosen your body by moving your arms and legs around slowly and naturally – twist your ankles and wrists from side to side and pivot your neck. This will relieve any minor pent up muscle tension you may possess and cause blood circulation to increase throughout your entire body.

Once this is accomplished, sit down in Lotus Posture on the floor. As discussed, if the cross-legged posture is uncomfortable, you can preform this exercise by sitting with your spine erect in a chair.

Once you have settled into your seated posture, close your eyes and become comfortable with your body. What this entails is to simply mentally relax into your positioning.

Sitting Consciously

Many people sit down with the intention of immediately entering into a meditative *Chi Kung* technique and attempt to mentally force themselves immediately into the exercise. What this does is cause your adrenal gland to release hormones, which causes your heart rate to increase and your mind to become alerted, and active. This is the exact opposite of what you wish to achieve in this exercise. Therefore, never force yourself to sit down and expect to immediately enter into a meditative mindset. Instead, take a few moments to become comfortable with your positioning.

Once you feel that you are mentally ready, consciously take in a very deep breath through your nose – feel your lungs and stomach expand with the inhalation. This inhalation should not be unnaturally forced, but should, none-the-less, cause your lungs to fill completely, thereby, expanding your chest and stomach. Once your in-breath is completed, the Chi filled oxygen should be allowed to leave your lungs naturally, exiting through your mouth.

Perform this deep breathing exercise by taking air in through your nose and allowing it to be exhaled through your mouth for seven complete breath cycles.

Deep Breathing

Deep breathing is one of the most basic and fundamental things you can do to not only instantly revitalize yourself with Chi but to cleanse your lungs from the pollutants of the modern world. The initial deep inhalation of new air in the *Tiao Chi* exercise, additionally, performs the task of cleansing the body's Meridian pathways. This is accomplished because of the fact that the human body is in a constant pattern of taking in vital Chi through the breath in the same rhythmic pattern hour after hour, day after day. Throughout your life you breathe in a constant pattern, thus, your body becomes accustomed to a specific level of Chi entering your being with each breath cycle. By inhaling deeply, you instantly change this pattern and your body becomes alive with excessive amounts of Chi. What naturally occurs from this process is that your Meridian pathways are instantaneously purged from any blockage which may have resulted from the stagnation of Chi.

Tiao Chi: Exercise Two

Upon the completion of the initial stage of *Tiao Chi* you will want to immediately continue forward with the second stage of this exercise, which witnesses you focusing your meditative attention upon your breath. To do this is quite simple. Breathe calmly in through your nose. As the breath enters your body, witness its life giving force traveling naturally through your nose, down into your lungs. When it is time to exhale, do so naturally through your mouth.

At this stage of *Chi Kung* no element of your breath is forced or controlled. You simply observe the Chi filled energy of life naturally entering and exiting your body. The breath comes in, it goes out -- you come to realize that you are only an earthly conduit for this divine process of Chi transmission.

A new breath comes in. You witness it. It goes out. You witness it. Allow yourself to simply *be.*

Perform this phase of the exercise for as long as you feel naturally inclined. As it is a very focusing and meditative process, it should go on for at least seven natural breath cycles, but can go on for much longer.

Once you have completed this stage of *Tiao Chi* you can move forward with additional *Chi Kung* exercises or simply encounter the day in a much more profoundly aware fashion.

4 Dan Tien

In Chinese, the term *Dan Tien* means, *"Field of Elixir."*

Dan Tien is a term coined by ancient Taoist monks to describe the most important location on the human body in relation to conscious interaction with Chi.

This understanding has been adopted and used by many facets of Asian culture. To the acupuncturist this location is designated by the expression, *Quhai,* which is translated as, *"Sea of Chi."* In the Korean language it is named, *Tan Jun.* And, in Japanese the word *Hara* is used to defines this same bodily location.

The term *Hara* is perhaps the word that is most commonly known when describing this location on the human body. This is due to that fact of its frequent usage in association with Aikido and the Japanese Martial Arts in general.

Understanding Dan Tien

Dan Tien is the location on the human body where Chi congregates and can be accessed and utilized by the individual. Thus, this location is highly revered.

It is an absolute necessity that you become acutely aware of this bodily location in order that you may become consciously interactive with Chi. Thus, your first step in active *Chi Kung* is to become interactive with your *Dan Tien*.

Defining Dan Tien

Dan Tien is located approximately two inches below your naval. From a central point it goes out approximately two inches in each direction.

In addition to being the location where Chi congregates in your body, it is your body's center of gravity. For this reason, Martial Artists become highly aware of this energy center through practicing their advanced form of movement. In fact, whenever you hear a *Martial Artist* let out a yell, as they unleash a technique, it is signifying that they are releasing Chi energy in association with their movement.

Martial Artists are not the only individuals who can become sharply aware of their *Dan Tien*. This knowledge is available to anyone who places the proper focus upon this energy center.

To achieve this interactive knowledge you must initially perform a few simple movements which will help you define this bodily location. From this, you can move forward with *Chi Kung* and consciously bring Chi into all the movements of your everyday life.

Dan Tien Defining: Exercise One

Begin by standing in a natural position with your arm loosely down to your side. Keep your spine erect, but not stiff. Move your neck around a little bit, releasing any tension. Do the same with your shoulder.

When you feel comfortable, close your eyes. Slowly become very conscious of your body. This process should not be forced. Do not attempt to strain your mind, telling yourself, *"Be conscious – be conscious."* As you progress through several sessions with this exercise and other *Chi Kung* techniques, which are presented in this book, you will come to a state of refined interactive consciousness with your body. You will find that it is be a very natural process to become intuitively focused upon specific components of your being. Therefore, at the early states of your *Chi Kung,* never force your body or mind – simply begin to develop your new interrelationship with your body.

Body Consciousness

If this is your first endeavour into body consciousness, simply begin to take notice of how your body feels. First place your concentration on your feet. *"How do they feel?"* Then your legs... Move up to your torso, consciously taken notice of each inch of your body. Experience your arms, and finally your neck and head.

At the point you have taken inventory of all of these bodily locations, begin to focus your concentration upon the approximate location of your *Dan Tien*. Begin by mentally surveying this area of your body – a location that you have probably placed very little focus upon previously.

As the exact location of *Dan Tien* is unique to each individual, it is you who must locate *Dan Tien* on your own body. Thus, simply begin to mentally feel this region.

As your consciousness becomes more focused on this energy center, begin to witness your breath coming in through your nose. Feel it enter your body, providing you with life substantiating oxygen. Then, witness it exiting your body through your mouth. Do this for a few natural breath cycles and then begin to mentally send your breaths to your *Dan Tien* – visualize each in-breath traveling through your nose, deep into your body, and lighting up your *Dan Tien* with golden Chi filled energy.

Do not elongate these breaths for an unnatural period of time. Simply allow them to travel in and out of your body naturally. Each breath enters, touches your *Dan Tien* with golden Chi filled energy and then exits via your mouth.

After you have performed this segment of the exercise for approximately seven natural breath cycles – with your next in breath, again, watch it travel to your *Dan Tien*. Once this in-breath has been completed, hold it locked into your *Dan Tien* for approximately seven seconds. Then, release it naturally through your mouth. Do this segment of the exercise for approximately seven natural breath cycles and then return to normal breathing for a few minutes before you open your eyes and finish this exercise.

With the practice of this simple technique, you are consciously causing Chi energy to activate in your *Dan Tien*. From this, you will begin to develop an understanding of this vital energy center.

Dan Tien Defining: Exercise Two

Begin by standing in a natural stance as you did with *Dan Tien Defining Exercise One*. Loosen your body up and settle into a focused mental state with your eyes closed. Breathe naturally, consciously experience golden Chi filled breaths entering and invigorating your body.

When you feel that you are mentally ready, focus your attention on the area of your *Dan Tien* and begin to witness your breaths traveling to and from this energy center via your nose. After approximately seven natural breath cycles, bend your elbows bring your hands up to your waist level at the frontal region of your body. As you do, allow the inner tips of your fingers to come into light contact with your thumb.

In acupuncture it is understood that several Meridians culminate in the tips of your fingers. By joining your fingers and thumb together in this fashion, you seal off any Chi that may be randomly exiting your body. Thus, you maintain a more constant circulation.

As your next breath is taken in, witness it entering your body through your nose and traveling to your *Dan Tien* in a golden light. As it flows inward, allow your knees to lightly bend. In association with this bending, simultaneously pull your hands back at waste level until they reach your mid-side region as your in-breath is completed.

Hold this Chi breath in your body for approximately seven seconds, as you visualize the golden light of Chi energy emanating from your *Dan Tien,* expanding forward in front of your body.

When it is time to exhale, do so slowly. As your breath exits you body via your mouth, see it illuminating the area around your body in the form of golden Chi filled light. As you exhale, simultaneously bring your knees and your hands slowly back to their original positioning. When your breath has been completely exhaled, do not breathe in for approximately seven seconds. Instead, experience the lightness of Chi filled energy your body is experiencing.

After this interval, again breath in your Chi filled breath, as your body slowly lowers and your hands pull back, exposing your *Dan Tien* that is emanating Chi from this powerful energy center.

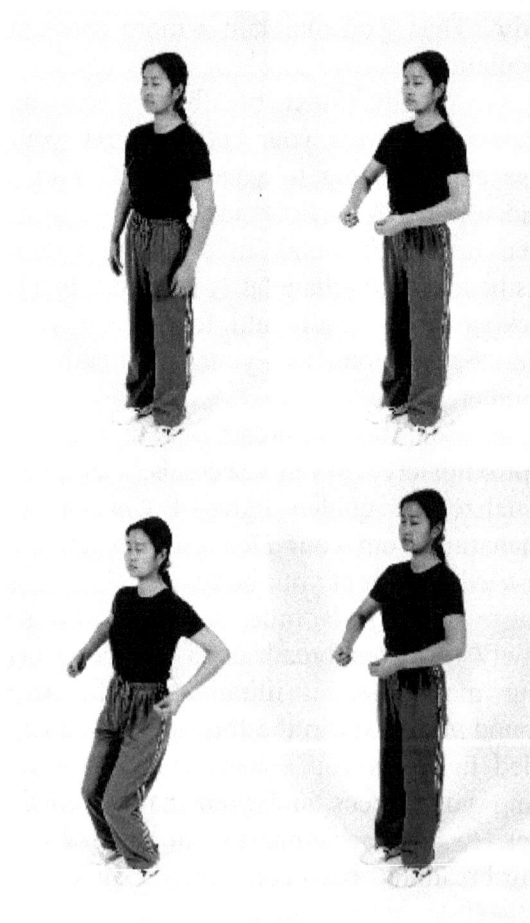

This exercise should be performed for a maximum of seven cycles per training session. From this, you will not only come to effectively define the exact location of your *Dan Tien* but you will additionally begin to experience how Chi can be brought into your body and then projected into the environment around you.

The Three Dan Tien

To the modern practitioner of *Chi Kung,* there is a single focal point that is the primary focus of Chi interaction, the *Dan Tien.* In ancient times, however, there were, in fact, three *Dan Tiens* that were accessed by the *Chi Kung* practitioner. This understanding was known as *San Dan Tien,* or the, *"Three Fields of Cultivation."*

The first of these three *Dan Tien* is the primary focal point detailed previously. From ancient times forward it has been known that this *Dan Tien* was the location in the human body where Chi energy congregated and could be drawn upon in times of need.

The second, or middle *Dan Tien,* known in Chinese as, *"Zhong Dan Tien,"* is located at the solar plexus. This energy center was believed to be responsible for proper breathing. An individual who focused his Chi orientated meditation upon this *Dan Tien* was believed to possess superior strength and unequalled endurance.

The third of these three energy centers is the *Zuigao* or the *"Upper Dan Tien."* This focal point is located at the pineal gland, commonly called, *The Third Eye.* Chi meditation upon this *Dan Tien* was known to provide the individual with superior mental skills.

Though the primary focal point for the *Chi Kung* practitioner is the *Dan Tien* located just below the navel, the two additional *Dan Tiens* are important energy centers which can be cultivated to access specific types of Chi. Therefore, these bodily locations must be embraced for the student of *Chi Kung* to come to an overall mastery of this science.

In the pages that follow, Chi Kung techniques which activate all three of the Dan Tiens will we detailed.

5 Tao Yin

Tao Yin, literally translated from the Chinese means, *"Stretching and Contracting the Body."* In practice, *Tao Yin* is the technique of performing seven ancient exercises that dissipate Chi obstructions from your body.

From ancient times forward, *Tao Yin* has been understood to not only invigorate the body with Chi but to prolong life and promise immortality. This is due to the fact that the seven exercises relieve the body of illnesses while invigorating it with Chi.

Tao Yin is additionally understood to focus the mind of the practitioner to the degree where the advanced techniques of Chi breath control and meditation can by mastered by the zealot.

Tao Yin is made up of highly exacting Chi purification techniques. The seven exercises that make up *Tao Yin* must be performed in a continual sequence, in order that all Meridians of your body are stimulated and cleared of any potential blockage.

When the seven *Tao Yin* exercises are performed, the intake and exhalation of breath must be implemented in an acutely focused manner. You cannot allow the physical aspects of your body's movement, in association with these exercises, to overpower your mental intent or the process of Chi infusion will not be actualized.

Tao Yin: Exercise One – Kou Ch'ih

Kou Ch'ih, translated from the Chinese, means, *"Chattering of the Teeth."* *Kou Ch'ih*, is not only the primary *Tao Yin* exercise but it is the preliminary exercise which, in ancient times, was performed before all *Chi Kung* techniques, due to its ability to nurture the brain and the body with necessary internal nutrients.

To correctly perform *Kou Ch'ih*, begin by closing your eyes and consciously encountering the vast abyss that exists in your own mental darkness. Mindfully embrace the understanding that within your own being is the link to divine consciousness and the darkness that you see should not be feared for it is a pathway to self discovery, where you can not only discover your meditative mind but *Ming*, *"Enlightenment,"* as well.

Once your eyes are closed, take a few moments to engage the darkness. When you feel it is time, place your mental focus on your breath and begin to breathe slowly and naturally for seven cycles – inhaling and exhaling through your nose. Feel the life giving breath entering and exiting your body.

Do not force your breath or mentally send it to any location within your body, simply observe the cosmic perfection of this process as your diaphragm expands with each in breath, filling your lungs with life giving oxygen and Chi and contracting with each out breath, leaving you with a sense of fulfilled lightness.

Upon the exhalation of the seventh breath, consciously direct all of the remaining air out of your lungs, allowing them to become completely empty. Accomplish this by contracting your upper abdomen muscles. Witness the feeling you experience as the final Chi filled breath exits your body through your mouth – leaving your being embraced in Chi saturated lightness.

Do not immediately breathe in again but begin to lightly bring your teeth together. Do not grind them or smash them upon one another, simply gently expand your jaw, with your lips remaining closed, and bring your upper teeth down upon your bottom teeth thirty-six times.

At first, the lack of air in your lungs may cause you emotional discomfort. If you must breathe during the thirty-six teeth chattering, do so calmly and naturally through your nose.

No Chi refining technique should cause you physical or emotional discomfort. This is especially the case with the exercise that makes up *Tao Yin*. Therefore, do not force any exercise, if you need to breathe, move, or reposition yourself to regain you physical or mental comfort, do so without hesitation.

As you move forward with *Chi Kung* techniques, it will become more and more natural for your lungs to remain absent of oxygen for extended periods of time. This is due to the fact that as you become increasingly filled with expanded amounts of Chi, you will learn to gain mastery over the repetitive elements of your physical being and they will no longer be seen as such a dominate factor of your existence.

While practicing *Kou Ch'ih* you should also not attempt to rush through the thirty-six movements of teeth chattering in order to breathe again, as this disrupts the meditative focusing involved in this Chi exercise. Simply allow your teeth to meet each other thirty-six times in a constant and paced pattern.

Upon the completion of the thirty-sixth *Teeth Chattering,* breathe in slowly and naturally through your nose. Experience the power of this Chi filled breath embracing your being.

Seated Kou Ch'ih

Kou Ch'ih is ideally practiced in a seated posture when it is used as a primary Chi focusing technique prior to additional seated *Chi Kung* techniques. When it is used in association with the other six *Tao Yin* exercises, however, it is more appropriately performed from a standing position. This is due to the fact that six of the seven *Tao Yin* exercises are dependent upon a standing posture. Thus, it is much more conducive to the constant flow of Chi to not sit and then rise between these practices.

Standing Kou Ch'ih

To perform Kou Ch'ih from a standing posture, simply stand with your feet naturally separated at shoulder level. Your arms should be loosely at your side. Then simply perform the *Teeth Chattering* as described.

Kou Ch'ih and Yu Chiang

The ancient practice of *Kou Ch'ih* was designed to stimulate the body's production of *Yu Chiang, "Saliva."* To the Taoist, saliva is known as, *"Liquid Jade."* From a physiological standpoint saliva is believed to be one of the most nourishing elements produced internally within the human body. It is believed to feed the brain and moisten the *Wu Tsang, "The Five Organs:"* lungs, heart, pancreas, kidneys, and liver. It is understood that spitting is one of the worst things an individual can do, because this unnecessarily wastes this vital liquid from the body.

Tun To

Upon the completion of *Kou Ch'ih,* the saliva that has been produced should be circulated around the mouth. Once this has been accomplished, *Tun To* is performed. *Tun To* is the ancient Taoist Chi practice of slowly and consciously swallowing the saliva, thereby, fostering the continued health of the body and allowing Chi to move freely within it.

Ancient Traditions – Modern Science

To the modern individual, the thought that saliva is a nurturing element to the whole of the human being is often times immediately dismissed as ancient superstition. When one takes on the practice of *Chi Kung,* however, they rapidly come to understand, through experience, that though some of the techniques may be rooted in timeworn traditions, the physical and mental exhilaration which occurs from them instantly provides one with the insight that though modern science may provide clearer physiological definitions of biological actions, the ancient Chi development exercises prove that energy is, in fact, developed and cultivated when the techniques are put into practice.

To this end, it is imperative to never simply dismiss any ancient Taoist *Chi Kung* technique, simply because it may seem somewhat absurd based in modern scientific analysis. Though these practices may be thousands of years old, they would not have continued to be utilized had they not provided results. Therefore, with personal exploration and performance, you will experience that each step of each application fills you with the empowerment of Chi.

Tao Yin: Exercise Two

The second Tao Yin exercise is known as, *"The Ocean Churns as you Swallow its Essence."*

To perform this technique, stand in a loose and natural posture. Close your eyes and take in a few natural breaths, inhaling through your nose and exhaling through your mouth. Mentally witness these breaths traveling to and emanating from your *Dan Tien.*

After a few moments of *Dan Tien* breath meditation, begin to very consciously feel your body. Start at your feet. Is there any tension? If there is, move them slightly as you watch golden Chi traveling from your *Dan Tien* down your leg to embrace and revitalize them. Once you have performed this, place your feet firmly back upon the ground. Direct your consciousness to your ankles. If there is any discomfort, move them around slowly as you direct Chi to them. Move your consciousness up your legs, truly experiencing them. If you experience any lack of comfort, breathe Chi into them. Feel your hands. Any pressure? Move them slightly and send them Chi. Allow your consciousness to travel up your torso, feel you neck and head. If any bodily location is experiencing an uneasy feeling, move it slightly, causing added blood circulation, and then very consciously breathe Chi from your *Dan Tien* to that location.

Remember Chi is endless. All you need to do is breathe in its power and you will be reenergized.

Once you have become very consciously in tune with your body, *"Ocean churns as you swallow its essence,"* continues by taking in a deep breath through your nose and watching it travel to your *Dan Tien* in a gold flow. Once the breath has completely entered your Dan Tien, you hold it in place and begin to circulate your tongue around your closed mouth ten times. At the completion of the tenth cycle, place your tongue firmly against your palate and release the gold breath of Chi through your nose. Witness it encompassing your body.

You will have witnessed that excess saliva is being produced in your mouth. When it is time to breath again, do so naturally, bringing the breath in through your nose. As the in-breath is completed, allow this excess saliva to be slowly swallowed nourishing your entire being. It will take approximately three natural breath cycles to consciously performed this *Tun To* exercise.

By performing this third element of the *Tao Yin* you will have accomplished *Tai Shih* or, *"Feeding of the Embryo."* This expression details that your inner being is flushed with Chi.

Tao Yin: Exercise Three

The third stage of *Tao Yin* is known as, *"Turning the Heavenly Pillar."* To begin this exercise, leave your eyes closed and consciously take in one deep breath through your nose. Witness this breath traveling to your *Dan Tien* and filling it with golden Chi energy. Lock this breath in this positioning for a moment, embracing its power. When you feel that it is necessary, naturally release this Chi breath through your mouth. With your next in-breath, taken in through your nose, guide it towards your *Dan Tien,* open your eyes, bring your palms together in front of you body, with your left hand facing upwards, your right hand facing downward – allow them to meet just in front of your solar plexus. Leave your feet in a stationary position, pointing naturally forward, and turn your upper torso towards the right from waist level. As you reach your maximum pivot, while keeping your spine erect, guide your shoulders a little farther to the right than is natural for you. Consciously embrace this upper body stretch.

As this movement is performed, allow your eyes to look as far to your left as is possible without actually moving your head. When it comes time to release your in-breath, do so, bringing your body and eyes back to their natural central positioning.

With your next natural in-breath, turn your body in the same fashion to the left, allowing your eyes to look extremely to the right. Release the breath when it is time and return to your central position. This movement should be performed seven times in association with each new in-breath.

The purpose of this exercise, from a physical standpoint, is to stimulate your Meridian pathways through a technique of movement that is natural, yet slightly exaggerated. From a more metaphysical perspective, this exercise moves the body in one direction, while the eyes and their vision travel in the opposite. What this serves to symbolize is that within all *Yang* this is the element of *Yin* – as within all *Yin* there is *Yang*. Your two hands remain touching one another to center and intermingle the *Yin* and the *Yang,* thus grounding your being in the balance of the two primary energies of this universe.

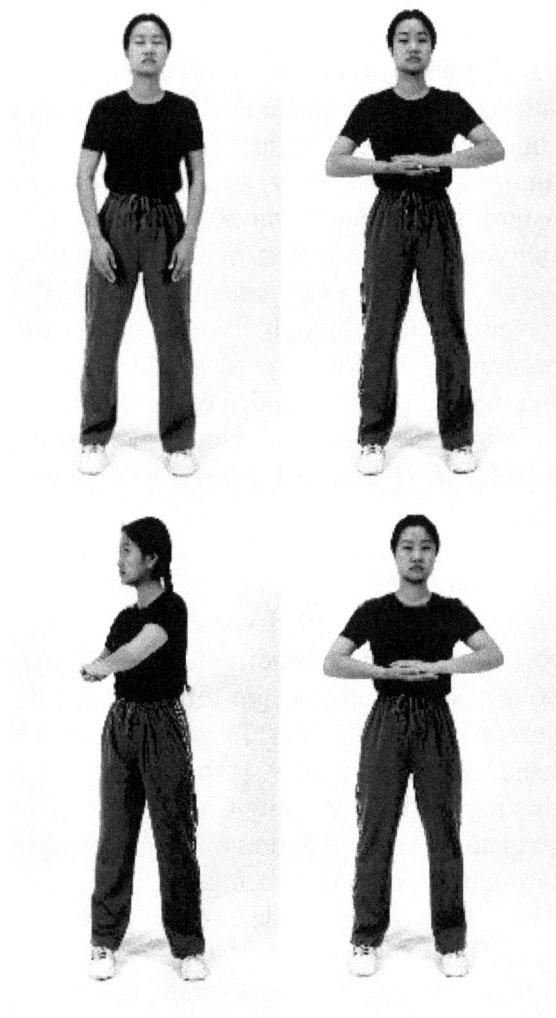

Tao Yin: Exercise Four

Tao Yin exercise four begins by you rubbing your hands together to make them warm from the friction. Do not simply allow them to warm with no consciousness of what is actually taking place. As all Chi development exercises are based in mental science, you must make all *Chi Kung* a very conscious process of mental evolution. To this end, close your eyes and breathe naturally in through your nose as you gently rub your hands together. With each new in-breath visualize the golden light of Chi traveling in through your nose and progressing to your hands, as they become illuminated with the golden essence of Chi.

At the point your hands have become warm and invigorated with Chi, generally after three to five breath cycles, place your left hand on your *Dan Tien* and your right hand on your forehead. For a moment, embrace the Chi filled warmth your hands reveal upon these bodily locations. With your next in-breath, begin to lightly rub the area around your *Dan Tien* with your left hand. Experience how your hand rubbing this region dissipates any Chi which may be stagnating and witness it expanding throughout your entire being.

When one single in-breath and out-breath have been completed, cease your rubbing action. Take one more natural in-breath in through your nose, feel it expand your lungs with Chi filled air. Allow this breath to naturally leave your body through your nose.

With your next in-breath, begin to rub your forehead – experience how the Chi energy locked in your *Third Eye, "Zuigao"* is released throughout your body. At the completion of one natural in-breath and one natural out-breath, allow both of your hands to return to natural positions on your side. Take a few moments for natural breathing, experiencing the Chi radiating throughout your body.

See page 82

Tao Yin: Exercise Five

With your eyes remaining closed, bring your consciousness to your breath and progress through three natural breath cycles – witness golden Chi traveling to your *Dan Tien* and radiating throughout your body from this location. When you have completed the third exaltation, bring your hands together and again, in association with your Chi conscious breath, rub them together in front of you until they are suitably warmed up. When you have completed this process, bring your hands around your back and place them upon your kidney region.

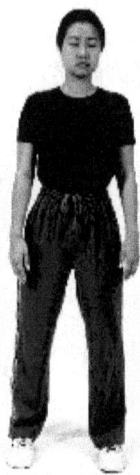 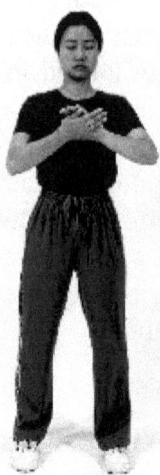

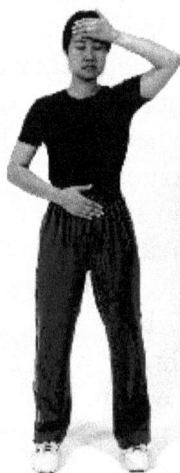 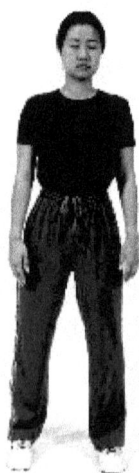

As your kidneys are elementally important organs to the proper functioning of your human body and are understood to be very important in the proper circulation of Chi, they too must be freed from any potential obstructions, so that Chi can flow unhindered throughout your being. With your warm hands, rub them in an up and down motion thirty-six times in the kidney region of your back. Breathe naturally as you witness with each in-breath golden Chi flowing in through your nose, traveling down your arms and embracing your kidneys with the freeing energy of golden Chi light. Exhale each out-breath via your mouth.

When you have completed this procedure, bring your hands back to your side, breathe naturally and embrace the continually evolving freedom your ethereal body is encountering.

See page 84

Tao Yin: Exercise Six

After a few moments of meditative reflection upon completion of *Tao Yin, Exercise Five,* again, bring your consciousness to your breath, breathe in Chi though your nose, and send it down your arms as you rub your hands together for a third time.

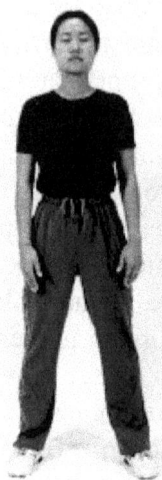 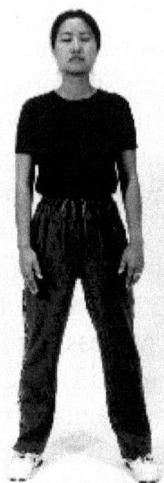

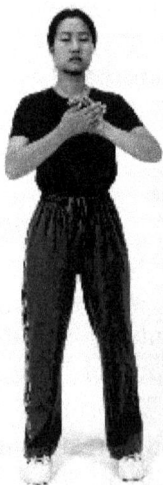 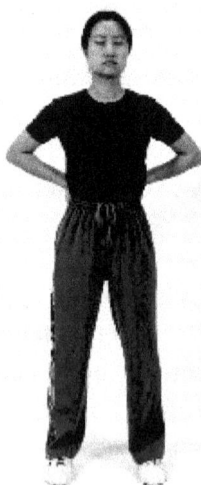

Once they are suitably filled with Chi, place your warm hands on the back of your head, with your palms covering your ears. Allow your fingers to extend around the back of your skull. Focus your consciousness on your breath as you breathe in a natural and deep Chi filled breath through your nose. When the in-breath is complete, lock it in your *Dan Tien*. At the same time, begin to lightly tap your forefingers on the rear of your skull, close to your spine. This tapping should be performed for a total of thirty-six repetitions, thus, relieving any Chi blockage that may have occurred along your spine and in your cranium.

Upon the completion of the thirty-sixth tap, return your hands to your side and meditatively breathe naturally.

See page 86 & 87

Your Hands and Tao Yin

The Chi filled rubbing of your hands in *Tao Yin* is performed in order that you very consciously send Chi to your hands. This is done in order for you to help in the removal of Meridian blockages that may have occurred in your body. The same techniques of *Tao Yin* that you perform on your own body can additionally be used when you are going to perform acupressure or massage another individual to aid in the removal of Chi blockage in their body.

Therefore, the techniques of *Tao Yin* are not only beneficial to enhanced Chi flow throughout your body but can additionally be beneficial to other human beings, as well.

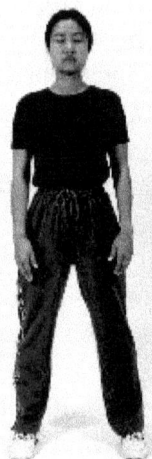

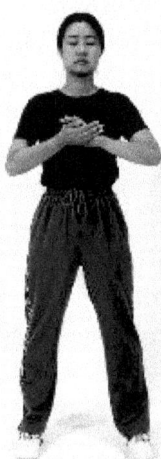

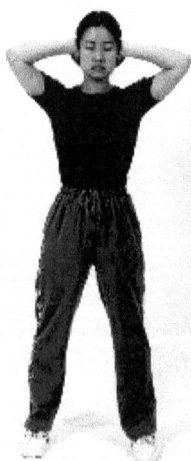

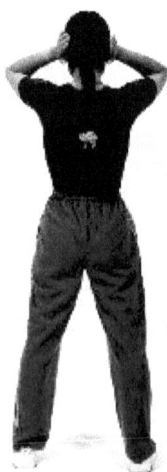

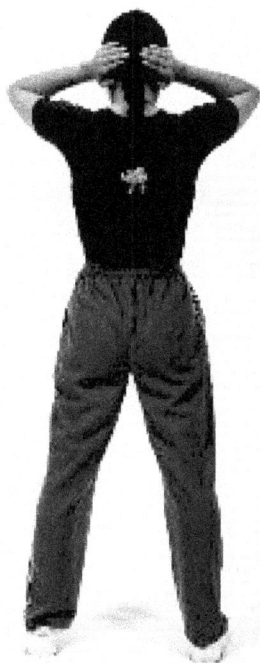

Tao Yin: Exercise Seven

Your eyes remain closed as you progress into the seventh stage of *Tao Yin,* known as, *"Bringing in the Double Wind."* As your common Chi blockage locations have been freed by this point in your *Tao Yin* experience, it has therefore become much easier for you to successfully bring excess amounts of Chi into your body and have it flow unhindered. Thus, it is now time to not only clear any final blockage points, but to invigorate your entire physical being and surroundings with positive Chi energy.

Begin by breathing a few natural breath cycles. When you feel you are ready, consciously exhale. As you do so, extend your arms to their full length, parallel to the ground, in front of your body. Your hands should be open and your palms facing one another at approximately a one-foot separation. When it is time for you to inhale, do so powerfully, with focused determination. As this Chi breath enters your body, through your nose, see it dynamically traveling to your *Dan Tien*. As your breath comes in, simultaneously make your hands into fists and draw them towards you as if you were pulling a heavy object into your body.

With the completion of your in-breath, feel the power of Chi emanating from your *Dan Tien* and physically enhancing your physical being and the external space around you.

Embrace this Chi power as you slowly mentally count to ten. Upon the tenth count, release this breath through your mouth, as your fists release and your arms travel outwards towards their original extended positioning. Once they have reached this level, allow your lungs to remain consciously empty for the same count of ten. Experience how your body is surging with Chi energy and your surroundings are vibrating with the Chi energy that emanated from your body.

At the count of ten, again breathe in Chi filled air as you perform this technique for a second time – making your hands into fists as they pull that large object towards your body and your entire being becomes filled with Chi. Once this action has been completed, again, count to ten and release the breath in the same pattern.

Tao Yin Seven should be performed a maximum of seven times. If you perform it more than seven times, your blood pressure has the potential to rise to an unacceptable level and you will defeat the purpose of this Tao Yin by causing your body to fall out of a natural balance.

Tao Yin and You

As you will experience from continued practice, *Tao Yin* is a process of not only cleansing the body of Chi blockage but it is a powerful meditation tool, as well. As you become more and more in tune with your body, when you perform this exercise, you will come to feel blockage points free up during the techniques. In addition, you will begin to very consciously experience Chi travel throughout your body, not only making you more virile but immensely more healthy, as well.

6 Jin Guang

Jin Guang means, *"Golden Light."*
This is a *Chi Kung* meditation technique
which not only trains your thinking mind to
acutely focus but also invigorates your body
with Chi energy while revitalizing your
immune system.

Jin Guang Exercise: Part One

To perform *Jin Guang,* sit either in
cross-legged *Lotus Posture* on the floor or in
a chair with your spine erect. Completely
close your eyes and naturally observe your
breath for a few moments as you allow your
mind to calm.

Once you have suitably centered
yourself, open your eyes just slightly. Place
your vision's focus upon the end of your
nose. Once you have located this
positioning, begin a cycle of eleven natural
breaths. Allow these breaths to slowly enter
through your nose and exit via your mouth.

Do not force these breaths. As each
one enters your body through your nose,
visualize the golden light of positive Chi
energy enter and revitalizing all elements of
your physical and spiritual being. As each
breath exits your body, mentally see all of
your negativity, anger, and impurities exiting

your body in the form of charcoal colored smoke.

When you have completed the cycle of eleven natural Chi breaths, close your eyes. Allow your mental focus to encompass your entire being. Feel how revitalized you are – how refreshed you feel due to the expelling of all negativity, while you refreshed yourself with the positive force of Chi.

Jin Guang Exercise: Part One
Second Segment

After a few moments of mental reflection, again, place your visual focus upon the tip of your nose – perform another cycle of eleven Chi filled breaths. This time, as you inhale through your nose, feel the golden Chi energy filling your being with positive Chi energy. As you exhale through your mouth, visualize this golden light emanating from your body and encompassing your entire being with positive strength, and goodness.

The process of *Jin Guang* not only permeates your being with positive Chi energy as you practice this *Chi Kung,* but it is an on-going and expansive exercise. You will find that after you have performed this *Chi Kung* for a time, your body will become such a conduit for positive Chi energy that you will be able to extend your positive Chi further and further. It will embrace the room where this technique is practiced, the building where you find yourself, and finally the entire world.

Meditation Remembrance

It is important to remember that *Chi Kung* meditation is not a selfish practice. It is for this reason that in this elementary technique your eyes remain slightly opened. From this, you achieve a meditative state of awareness, while remaining connected to the external world.

Sharing Your Chi

Meditation focuses the mind, thereby refining the energy in each human being. This is especially the case with *Chi Kung* orientated meditation techniques.

When you begin to meditate, you should not do it solely as a means to enhance your own physical and mental state of well-being. It is imperative to take the positive energy developed in *Chi Kung* and share it with the world. By living your life in this fashion you not only gain meditative insight, but you will continually encounter only the most positive of people and life situations as you are consciously adding to the overall positive energy of this physical plane of existence we have named the Earth.

Jin Guang Exercise: Part Two

The Second Segment of *Jin Guang* witness you unite golden spheres of light in two important energy centers within your body. The segment can only be performed after the first part of *Jin Guang* has been completed because your body must be initially cleared of negative energy – as negativity hinders the movement of Chi.

To perform *Jin Guang Part Two* remain seated, close your eyes, breathe calmly and naturally through your nose for a few moments. When you feel that you have become centered, begin the second level of *Jin Guang* by taking a deep breath in though your nose. Allow the golden Chi energy of this breath to travel to your *Dan Tien.* Once the in-breath has been completed, witness its Chi energy form a golden ball of Chi light in your *Dan Tien.* Hold this breath for a few moments longer than is natural, as this mental image becomes clear in your mind.

Embrace the ball of Chi light. Then release this breath of empowerment through your mouth. Allow your lungs to become completely empty as you continue to hold your mental focus upon the golden sphere of light in the *Dan Tien.*

Do not concentrate on your absence of breath. Instead, see and feel this golden ball of Chi light empowering this sacred bodily location.

When you feel it is time to breathe again – physically breathe in through your nose but mentally see this breath entering your body through your *Zuigao, "Third eye."* With this new in-breath, send the golden light of Chi towards your pineal gland, which is known as the *Upper Dan Tien.*

The Pineal Gland
The pineal gland is a small organ in the brain. It is located above the cerebellum and is connected to the third ventricle of the brain in all vertebrate animals, of which we, as human being, are one. The pineal gland possesses extensive nerve fibers and is highly saturated with blood due to the large number of blood vessels that exist within it. In certain reptilian and amphibian creatures such as lizards, frogs, and some strain of fish, the pineal gland is the scientifically known location where the amount and the depth of light is sensed. Thus, it is understood to be *The Third Eye* of these species.
The presence and overall effects of the pineal gland on the human being is not completely understood by modern science. It is known that the gland produces the hormone melatonin and that the gland affects the body's biorhythms and biological clock.

From a metaphysical perspective the pineal gland has for centuries been understood to be the gland that is directly linked to the metaphysical third eye of the individual. *The Third Eye* is a highly revered bodily location as it links the physical body to the ethereal body via the pineal gland. Due to the fact, *The Third Eye* is one of the primary locations which one focuses upon during meditation.

At the outset of this *Chi Kung* exercise it may be initially difficult for you to know the exact physical placement of your pineal gland. Do not let this concern you. Simply allow the golden Chi filled breath enter your body through your third eye and travel to a central placement in your cranium. Witness the Chi from a golden ball of light in this location. Through this practice, the exact site of you pineal gland will eventually present itself and become very obvious, as your Chi energy will be drawn to it.

Once your have visualized this golden ball of light in your pineal gland and have embraced this Chi filled third eye breath for a natural amount of time. Mentally witness the breath exiting your body through your third eye. Feel its power encompassing your body and the area around your seated location.

In the moments before you take your next breath, mentally observe the golden balls of Chi light existing in your Dan Tien and your pineal gland. See them pulsate with the power of Chi.

When it is time to take your next breath, bring it in through your *Third Eye,* allow it to travel first to your pineal gland and then move down through your body linking to your Dan Tien. Feel the power of this Chi breath uniting these two sacred locations and empowering you with universal energy.

Hold this breath for a few moments longer than is natural and then release it. Watch as the golden Chi breath leaves your *Dan Tien,* passes through your pineal gland, and then exits your body through your third eye.

As with the previous *Jin Guang,* perform this exercise eleven times – uniting the two spheres of Chi. With each in-breath witness the golden power of Chi entering your body, leaving you with not only enhanced power but with sustained overall physical and mental health, as well.

When you have concluded the second segment of the Jin Guang exercise it is important not to jump up and go out and encounter the enormity of the physical world. Instead, take a few moments, consciously absorbing the power of Chi. Embrace the energy before you go out and tackle the world.

7 Yen Chi

Yen Chi translates from the Chinese into, *"Swallowing the Chi Breath."*

As is the case with many *Chi Kung* techniques, *Yen Chi* activates both the body and the mind of the practitioner. With a combination of body movement in association with conscious breathing, the practitioner is brought into a mindful harmony of physical and ethereal understanding.

The Importance of Yen Chi

Yen Chi is an elementally important developmental exercise in the practice of *Chi Kung.* This is because of the fact that it teaches the practitioner the methods of harnessing the Chi that is emanating from the *Dan Tien.*

The practice of *Yen Chi* details that the *Chi Kung* Practitioner brings a Chi filled breath deeply into their *Dan Tien.* Then, as it is released, what is known as *Nei Chi, "Inner Chi,"* is harnessed before it is allowed to escape from the body. From this, the student learns how to hold excess amount of Chi in the body to be used in times of physical and mental need.

Yen Chi Exercise

You can begin the *Yen Chi* exercise from where ever you are. In fact, once you have come to master this technique you will be able to utilize it whenever you are in need of rapid Chi replenishment of excess physical or mental strength.

As is the case with all *Chi Kung,* it is best to begin by performing *Tao Yin* to focus your body and mind. The *Yen Chi* exercise is no different.

When you feel that you are mentally prepared, begin by standing up in a natural posture. Loosen any tension in your body up by performing light movement. Close your eyes and begin to focus your attention upon your *Dan Tien.*

Watch your natural in-breaths travel from your nose to your *Dan Tien,* saturating this region with golden Chi light. As your breath travels out of your *Dan Tien,* see its golden presence illuminating your entire being as it is exhaled from your mouth.

Observe this Chi breath process for several natural breath cycles. When you begin to experience Chi empowerment, breathe in and hold the breath locked in your *Dan Tien* for approximately seven seconds. As you begin to release it, watch it travel up to your *Middle Dan Tien, "Zhong Dan Tien,"* at your solar plexus. At the moment it reaches this region, close your mouth locking it off. Allow this Chi breath to emanate its power in this region. Mentally see this energy center radiating with Chi.

Your next step will be to swallow this Chi filled breath back into your *Lower Dan Tien*. This is achieved by mentally observing the golden Chi filled energy being held in your *Middle Dan Tien*. Then, as you swallow, you mentally witness it traveling back to your *Lower Dan Tien*.

As discussed in *Tao Yin,* (Chapter 5), saliva is understood by the Taoist to be *"Liquid Jade,"* a very beneficial bodily element. Thus, what you are doing is causing the Chi you have brought in from the air around you to not be released but instead to be redirected back to your *Dan Tien* via *Liquid Jade.*

Once you have mentally witnessed the golden Chi re-enter your *Dan Tien,* you can release the breath, as its Chi has been harnessed.

As you begin the practice of *Yen Chi,* it may only be possible for you to perform this technique one time. This is fine, as your body will be invigorated with the Chi you have harnessed. As you progress with your *Chi Kung* understanding, you will develop the ability to bring in and harness as much Chi energy as will be necessary for any particular action you are about to undertake.

No Savings Account for Chi

It is an important fact to remember that there is no savings account for Chi. Chi is everywhere. As such, it must remain in constant motion. If you attempt to harness Chi for your own selfish reasoning, its energy will overpower you.

For this reason, you should only practice *Yen Chi* when you have a specific physical or mental task to accomplish. Bring the excess Chi into your being, utilize it and then allow it to flow free, again, stimulating the entire universe.

8 Pi Chi

Pi Chi means, *"Holding your Chi Breath."*

Pi Chi is the practice of consciously holding Chi filled breath in your body for a prolonged period of time. From the practice of *Pi Chi* it is believed that you develop the ability to heal injured areas of your body.

Your Heart and Pi Chi

The practice of *Pi Chi* brings you into close harmony with the heart. The reasoning for this is that as you perform this exercise you will be monitoring how long you are holding your breath by how many heartbeats have elapsed.

The majority of the world's populous is completely out of tune with their hearts. They certainly know that a organ known as the heart is present in their body, but they only take notice of it when it is beating fast due to excessive physical exertion or coronary disease. The *Chi Kung* practitioner, on the other hand, realizes that the heart is one of the most essential elements to life. Therefore, through exercises such as *Pi Chi* its function is brought highly into focus and they maintain a continued awareness of its essential value to life.

The Advanced Nature of Pi Chi

Due to the fact that *Pi Chi* involves the conscious retention of the breath, it is an advanced technique of *Chi Kung.* When a person who is not suitably trained in the methods of Chi breath retention attempts to hold their breath for an extended period of time, they not only cause the natural patterns of their body to be sent out of alignment, but they risk passing out due to lack of oxygen to their brain. For this reason, *Pi Chi* should only be practiced in its most elemental form until the *Chi Kung* practitioner has come, through experience, to master some of the more subtle levels of Chi breath understanding presented in *Tiao Chi* and *Yen Chi.*

The *Pi Chi* exercise can be performed from either a standing or seated positioning. Which ever one you choose, remember to keep your spine erect and your body free from unnecessary tension.

Pi Chi Exercise

Enter into a quiet environment, close your eyes, and allow thoughts to leave your mind. Begin to watch your breath naturally traveling into your body through your nose and exiting through you mouth. Witness each natural in-breath traveling to your *Dan Tien,* illuminating it with golden Chi energy.

After approximately seven natural breath cycles, allow your new in-breath to naturally travel into your *Dan Tien*. This time, instead of allowing it to naturally leave, consciously close your mouth and tighten up your nasal passageway as it begins to rise. Retrain this breath in your *Dan Tien*.

Begin to witness your heartbeat. Count how may beats go by before you must release your Chi breath and breathe in new life giving oxygen.

As detailed, at the outset, do not attempt to force yourself to hold the breath longer than is natural. You are not in any type of competition. Simply take in the breath, and mentally make a note of how many heartbeats go by as you hold it. For the average person, at the beginning stages of this exercise, it will probably be for approximately three to four heartbeats.

Perform this practice of retaining your breath in your *Dan Tien* for approximately seven breath cycles. Then, release the final breath and breathe naturally for several cycles bringing your respiration back to a normal pattern.

After a few moment of mental centering, begin to focus on any part of your body that may be injured, not feeling well, or simply a location where you may need extra Chi. For example, if you know you are going to be lifting heavy objects in the very near future, you can focus on your arms.

As you breathe in your next breath, direct it to the location on your body you have isolated. Mentally see the golden light of Chi traveling to that location: illuminating, healing, and giving strength to that region.

As you hold this healing Chi filled breath, again count your heart beats. When it is time to release, do so. Immediately, bring in a new Chi filled breath and direct it to that same bodily location.

This stage of the exercise should be performed for up to seven cycles at the beginning of your *Pi Chi* practice. As you become more proficient with it, this time period can be extended, as you feel necessary.

Location, Location, Location

It is essential that you do not direct Chi to first you arms, then your ankles, and then your back in any one *Pi Chi* session. This practice will disrupt the focusing of Chi energy to a specific region.

If you possess several areas that you wish to heal, you should focus on one at time. Then, allow a several hour interval before you address a secondary region. From this, the Chi you focus on each region will have the opportunity to revitalize the region and multiple focusing will not dissipate its healing energy.

Ancient Pi Chi

In ancient times it was believed that a person must be able to direct their Chi breath to a bodily location and hold it for a minimum of seven heartbeats to effect healing. The longer the retention, the more Chi healing which took place. As the *Chi Kung* practitioner developed further, it was believed that when they could hold their breath for a total of one thousand heartbeats, they were approaching immortality.

9 Nei Tan

Nei Tan, literally translated from Chinese, means, *"Inner Cinnabar."*

Cinnabar is a mercury ore believed by the ancient Taoist alchemist to possess qualities which, when properly harnessed, could lead one to immortality. The choice of this word allows the modern *Chi Kung* practitioner to understand the importance the ancient Taoists places upon this mineral.

Ancient Nei Tan

In its most ancient understanding, the practice of Nei Tan witnessed Taoist alchemists combine various herbs, minerals, and cinnabar in order to create a potion that they hoped would induce immortality. This mythical elixir was referred as, *"Chang Shen Pus Su."*

By the beginning of the Sung Dynasty (960-1279 C.E.), however, the various Taoist schools, having become highly influenced by Buddhism, left behind the belief that any elixir could provide them with immortality. They began to reevaluate their understanding of immortality and realized that the road to this sought after plateau was only obtainable via highly refined breath control and meditation techniques that would lead the practitioner to enlightenment. At the point the practitioner reached spiritual realization, and, as such, the unceasing wheel of cause and effect, known as *Karma* would no longer bind them. Thus, they would become spiritually immortal.

The Practice of Nei Tan

The schools that embraced *Nei Tan,* at this historic juncture, believed that the process to enlightenment began in meditation where the practitioner must become acutely attuned to their *Ching, "Essence."* Then, by practicing specific breath control purification techniques they could become one with their *Chi, "Internal Energy,"* By remaining pure and being one with Chi, the practitioner could continue on with breath control exercises and meditation eventually transforming their Chi into *Shen, "Pure Spirit."* With this accomplished, they could then enter into the final stage of self-purification, known as, *Lien Shen Fu Hsu* or *"Integrating the self with the universe."*

This final step could only be taken by one, who through advanced purification, returned to the ultimate state of nothingness, known in Chinese as, *"Wu."* Thus, achieving enlightenment and immortality.

Understanding Modern Nei Tan

Nei Tan has evolved into a precise Chi orientated breath control exercises whereby the *Chi Kung* practitioner causes Chi to rise up the spine and circulate through the entire body. This process, similar to the practices of *Kundalini Yoga,* provides the practitioner with not only an enhanced sense of energy and power but stimulates the Chi which is locked in the base of the spin, thus leading to an overall sense of euphoria. Many believe this stimulated energy is a direct pathway to enlightenment.

Nei Tan: Exercise One

Begin the practice of *Nei Tan* by performing the seven *Tao Yin* exercises, thereby, focusing your mind and stimulating your *Nei Chi, "Inner Chi."* Upon the completion of *Tao Yin,* move into a cross legged seated positioning. As is the case with all *Chi Kung,* the cross-legged *Lotus Posture* is best, but if you find this uncomfortable, then sitting in a chair with your spine erect can be substituted.

Once you are seated, close your eyes and observe your natural breathing process for several minutes. This will allow your internal energy to become accustomed to your seated posture. At the point you believe you are ready to proceed, bring in a deep Chi filled breath though your nose and mentally guide it to you *Dan Tien.* Visualize the golden light of Chi energizing your being as you hold this breath locked in place for a few moments. Release it through your mouth.

Tu Mai

Tu Mai is the Chinese expression that details the ascending pattern of energy that runs vertically up your spine. The *Nei Tan* exercise directly stimulates this ascending energy. Thus, to begin *Nei Tan* place your focus on the base of your spine.

When you are ready, strongly breathe in your next golden Chi breath and mentally direct it to the base of your spine. Hold this initial *Nei Tan* breath in place for approximately three seconds – as you experience its golden Chi energy vibrating in this bodily location. When you release it, do so by contracting the muscles in the area of your *Dan Tien* just slightly. This will cause the breath to leave your body more quickly than normal.

Dan Tien Note:

As you advance in *Chi Kung* you will come to be acutely aware of your *Dan Tien*. Through time and your continued practice, you will begin to naturally contract the muscles surrounding your D*an Tien* when you intend to release excess amounts of Chi or when you are consciously directing Chi to a specific bodily location.

In the early stages this practice must be consciously undertaken. As time progresses, however, it will occur virtually without a thought.

Directing Chi Up Your Spine

With your Dan Tien muscles lightly contracted, mentally witness the golden Chi breath traveling up your spine, coming over the top of your head, and exiting via your nose. When your exhalation is complete, immediately take in another deep Chi filled breath through your nose and direct it to the base of your spine. Hold it for three seconds as you did before and then, with the aid of your stomach muscles, guide it up your spine, over the top of your head, and out via your nose. Immediately upon your complete exhalation, perform the process again.

The basic *Nei Tan* exercise should be performed for a maximum of seven cycles in the beginning stage of its practice. If you begin to feel light headed before this point, immediately stop.

Nei Tan: Exercise Two

At the point you have developed a foundational understanding of *Nei Tan,* you can move this technique to its advanced level. At this stage you consciously direct your Chi breath to activate specific bodily centers by causing Chi to transverse your body in a continuous circular flow.

It is important to note that you must be very conscious as you perform this exercise, as it is imperative that you do not let your mental focus slip or Chi may congregate in one of these bodily locations and ultimately stagnate. For this reason, the novice *Chi Kung* practitioner should only perform this technique for a maximum of three breath cycles in the early stages. As this is a very advanced form of *Chi Kung,* you must, through practice, have come to be truly interactive with Chi in order to truly understand and reap the benefits of this exercise.

The Eight Energy Centers

There are eight energy centers that will be consciously activated with this exercise.

They are:

1. *Dan Tien*

2. *Hai Di*

3. *Wei Lu*

4. *Ming Men*

5. *Nao Hu*

6. *Tein Len Gai*

7. *Su Liao*

8. *Shen Que*

The location of your *Dan Tien* should be well known to you by this point in your *Chi Kung* practice. Your *Hai Di* is located at the base of your groin. *Wei Lu* is at the base of your spine. *Ming Men* is located on your spine directly behind your heart. *Nao Hu* is on your spine at the base of the skull. *Tein Len Gai,* is the crown of your head. *Su Liao* is the tip of your nose. And finally, *Shen Que* is your naval.

If you study these bodily locations it can be easily understood why each is an essential active energy center. *Hai Di,* at the base of your groin is the center of creation. *Wei Lu,* at the base of your spine, is the energy center that is commonly understood to be the location of *Kundalini* or the Serpent Power. It is a bodily location where psychic power is based and awaits to be stimulated. In Chinese it is known as *Zhou Huo* or *"Fire Location."* *Ming Men* is located adjacent to your heart. It is the energy center that stimulates this essential organ. *Nao Hu,* at the base of your skull, is also known as, *"The Jade Pillow,"* or *"Yu Zhen."* This is your body's center of harmony with nature – for, if your spine is misaligned, Chi will not be allowed to flow throughout your being unhindered. *Tein Len*

Gai, crown of your head, is the source center for knowledge and intelligence. *Su Liao*, the tip of your nose, is your source point for conscious interaction with Chi, as it is where you physically bring Chi into your body. *Shen Que*, your naval, is the location of physical and spiritual nourishment, the source point for your life.

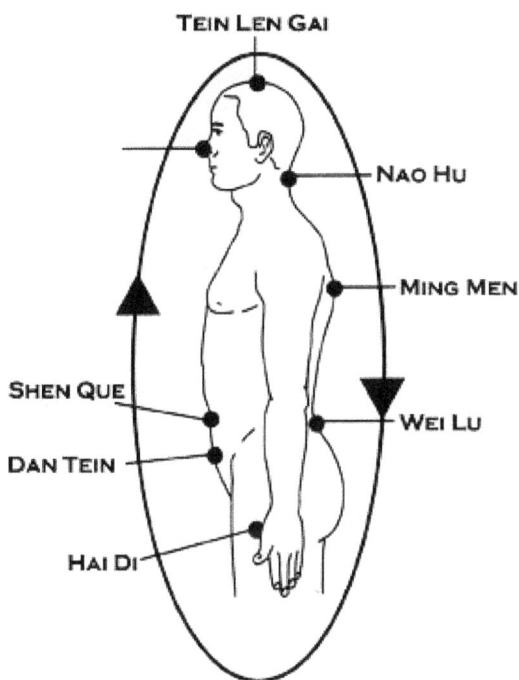

Beginning Nei Tan: Exercise Two

Now that you understand where your energy is to be directed, you can begin this exercise by sitting down in a cross-legged posture and calmly observe a few natural breaths enter and exit your body. When you feel focused, bring in a deep breath through your nose, send it to your *Dan Tien* and embrace its Chi. Completely release the breath after it has been held for approximately three heartbeats and consciously encounter the emptiness.

As you prepare to take your next in-breath focus on your *Dan Tien*. Breathe in the breath through your nose. As you do, witness a circle forming inside of your body, linking all of these energy centers. As your breath comes into your body, mentally see it entering this circular pathway. Witness it flowing in a nonstop fashion, illuminating each energy center as it passes through it. Allow the breath to exit via your mouth.

The process of the breath entering your body through your nose, revitalizing your energy centers, and then exiting your body via your mouth, should be timed to take place in a single, very conscious breath cycle. This advanced practice of exacting *Chi Kung* may take a little time for you to become accustomed to. Do not let this discourage you. Through practice, you will come to the point where you can control the intake of your breath to the degree that it passes through the energy centers and exits your body in a highly exacting fashion. From this mental coordination you will reach a new plateau in your *Chi Kung* understanding.

Once the breath has exited your body, embrace the emptiness for seven heartbeats as you witness your energy centers illuminated with power. As with all Chi Kung practices, if the full seven heartbeats are unnatural for you, take new breaths in when you feel you must.

The important thing to remember about this practice is that you must activate your energy centers with each in-breath. If you do not, the practice of *Nei Tan* will not provide results, as your breath-orientated conscious will come in and out of focus.

Nei Tan: Exercise Two should be practiced for a maximum of seven complete breath cycles in the beginning. As you become more and more proficient with your breath and energy center interaction, this technique can be performed for as long as you feel is appropriate.

The *Nei Tan* exercise is a very powerful technique which not only causes vast amounts of new Chi to rapidly infuse your being but it additionally stimulates Chi which may have remained dormant in your body for some time. For this reason, it is essential to remain very conscious while performing this technique. Never attempt to over do this exercise. Due to the amount of excess oxygen that is coming into your body, the novice can easily pass out.

10 Fu Jin Hsiang

Fu Jin Hsiang is the meditative practice of absorbing the Chi energy from the sun into your physical being.

It has long been scientifically documented that vegetation receives energy directly from the sun through the process known as photosynthesis. Human beings, though not elementally defined by a similar process, none-the-less, also draws vitamins and energy from the sun. This is especially the case when we consciously embrace the Chi energy of this life giving force.

Fu Jin Hsiang Exercise

The ancient Chinese practice of *Fu Jin Hsiang* witnesses the practitioner drawing the Chinese character for the sun, with a vermilion colored ink upon a rectangular shaped piece of green rice paper. For the modern practitioner, a simple image of the sun can be drawn onto a piece of green paper with red ink. Each morning the zealot then rises from sleep, sits on the floor in lotus posture, facing east, and places the paper in the left hand. The paper is clutched lightly as the practitioner practices the breathing exercise known as *"Breath of the Sun."*

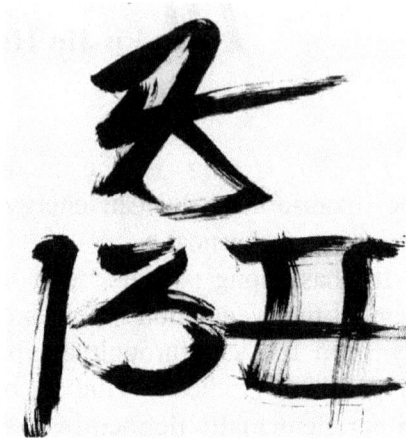

Breath of the Sun

To perform the Breath of the Sun, close your eyes and visualize a distant horizon with the red, orange, and yellow rays of the sun just beginning to crest over the darkened landscape. With your first breath, breathe in deeply as you witness your breath enters through your nose and traveling to your *Dan Tien* in an orange coloured flow of pure Chi energy. When you inhaliation is complete, hold the sun Chi breath in your *Dan Tien* for a moment and then release it.

Take your next in-breath as you mentally watch the sun slowly crest the horizon. Breathe in the suns energy. Witness it enter your body through the symbol of the sun you hold in your left hand. Watch this breath travel in a yellow, Chi filled flow, from your hand, through your arm, and onto your *Dan Tien*.

Hold this breath for a time; embrace its powerful presence. Then exhale through your nose. Witness the yellow Chi filled energy of the sun radiate throughout your being.

As you continue to breathe in sun Chi, mentally witness the sun slowly rise, completely over the horizon, feel its presence and power engulfing your being. Breathe in this power through your left hand and guide the energy to your *Dan Tien*. Hold it and then breathe out.

Fu Jin Hsiang should be practiced for up to a half an hour a day. As your sun mediation becomes deeper, you will be able to start with the sun below the horizon and then slowly watch it rise, culminating mid-sky in that half an hour period.

As you continue to practice this technique your being will become empowered with the sun's energy. You will be left feeling full of life and assured of your fortitude, determination, and your ability to overcome any obstacle.

The Sun and You

The mental visualization of the rising sun detailed in *Fu Jin Hsiang* exercise is the most applicable way for most modern practitioners to take part in this advanced Chi development technique. The ideal method to practicing this exercise, however, is to wake before the sun rises each morning and perform your Chi meditation in association with the actual sun cresting the horizon. In either case, it is essential that you truly embrace the Chi power of the sun for this exercise to lead you to an intimate interrelationship with sun Chi.

Sun Chi Meditation

This sun Chi exercise should be practiced as a meditation onto itself and not used in association with other advanced Chi meditation techniques. As in all Chi exercises you should begin with basic mental focusing techniques, but if you truly desire to be empowered with sun Chi you should not intermingle this meditation with other highly defined Chi focusing exercises, such as *Tao Yin,* or your focus will be dissipated and you will achieve noticeable results.

It is for this reason that ancient Taoist monks would choose one Chi meditation technique and focus solely upon it for a lifetime. From this style of highly defined practice, the ancient masters were born – possessing seemingly superhuman strength.

The Ancient Sun Masters

When the ancient practitioner of *Fu Jin Hsiang* would eventually achieve conscious interaction with *Sun Chi,* they would then dissolve the piece of rice paper which they used for their focus of meditation in a bowl of water and then drink it – substantiating their connection to *Sun Chi.*

For the modern application of this ancient exercise, once you have advanced to this level, you should very consciously take the paper and place it in an isolated compartment for a period of one year. If you were to simply throw it away, this will immediately dissipate your sun Chi. This is due to the fact that all objects of this universe possess energy. This is especially the case when an object has been used as a focus of meditation.

11 Lien Chi

Lien Chi, translated from Chinese, mean, *"Melting Chi Breath."*

Lien Chi is an ancient meditative breathing technique where Chi is allowed to flow unhindered throughout your entire body. Whereas many Chi breathing exercises guide Chi to a specific region of your body, for a exacting purpose, *Lien Chi* does not guide Chi to any specific Meridian, organ, or bodily location. Instead, its practice directs Chi to permeate your entire being – filling you with life revitalizing energy.

The Development of Lien Chi

The *Lien Chi* exercise was developed in ancient China. It was performed by Taoist sages who would dwell in mountain caves. It was believed that *Lien Chi* was the pathway to supernatural powers and immortality. This belief was based in the fact that from this exercise the body becomes permeated with Chi. Today, this technique is used as a meditative revitalizing exercise, which not only acutely focuses your mind but also renders your body charged with Chi.

Lien Chi – Advanced Chi Kung

Lien Chi is not an elementary Chi revitalizing exercise. It is performed only after the practitioner has gained substantial Chi understanding through the use of *Tiao Chi, Yen Chi,* and *Pi Chi* techniques.

Noise and the Lien Chi Exercise

The *Lien Chi* exercise is a very exacting form of *Chi Kung.* As such, when you perform this technique it is essential that you are not distracted by external noises. As many people live in urban environments, where soothing natural sounds are dramatically overpowered by the noises of the man-made world.

The random sounds of the physical world often times occur loudly and quickly. Thus, they can instantly jar you from your meditative consciousness. This type of rapid disruptive disturbance may cause your adrenal gland to release adrenaline. Once this occurs, your thinking mind will begin to travel rapidly from one thought to the next. If this transpires, it takes time to quiet and refocus your mind.

Due to the exacting nature of the *Lien Chi* exercise, if you are substantially disturbed, it is far better to simply change your focus and enter into contemplative meditation leaving this exercise for a later time rather than to try to regain the interrupted Chi energy experience of *Lien Chi.*

For these reasons, it may be necessary for you to take measures to ensure that you will not be distracted while practicing this technique. To this end, while performing *Lien Chi,* you can use earplugs or place cotton in your ears if you anticipate being distracted by the external world. Though this is certainly not the most beneficial way to perform this exercise, it is essentially important to not have your meditative mindset disturbed by external distraction.

Performing Lien Chi Exercise

Once you have entered a quite room and duly prepared for the exercise, remove all of your clothing. The reason your clothing is removed in *Lien Chi* is due to the fact that, not only does clothing restrict your body, but it also causes sensory perception to occur.

Clothing and Chi Kung

Take a moment right now, as you read this, and feel your body, which is more than likely clothed. No doubt, as you begin to focus, you can feel your clothing.

Throughout much of everyday life the sensation of actually wearing clothing is overpowered by the chaotic world, once you enter into refined Chi orientated meditation techniques, however, your senses become acutely turned to your physical being. For this reason, you must take every precaution to not be distracted from your focalization on Chi while you practice this exercise.

Preparing for Lien Chi

Once your clothes are removed, perform *Tao Yin* – focusing your body and mind, as you consciously come into contact with the universal energy of Chi. Once you have completed *Tao Yin* and your mind is relatively calm, lay down on your back.

As detailed in Chapter 2, the cross-legged *Lotus Posture* causes Chi to remain, *"Locked,"* in your upper torso. With *Lien Chi* you want Chi to permeate your entire body. For this reason, the laying posture allows it to flow throughout your being in the most unhindered pattern possible.

Laying Down

It is important that you do not lie on a bed or a couch. The reason for this is two-fold. First of all, these furniture items are generally not firmly supportive and your spine will have the tendency to relax into an unnatural positioning. Secondarily, beds and couches are commonly associated with rest and sleep. Thus, not only do they possess the vibration of relaxation but also your mind has been programmed into viewing these objects in that capacity. Therefore laying on the floor is mentally much more beneficial to the practice of *Lien Chi.*

If you have a hard wood or cement floor, lying on a rug or throw carpet, will keep you from becoming uncomfortable.

Lien Chi Exercise

Lay down on your back. Naturally extend your arms a few inches away from your torso. Allow your feet to be naturally separated – approximately two feet apart.

Begin by breathing naturally. Watch Chi filled air entering your body through your nose, providing you with the most essential element to life, oxygen.

Upon completion of your initial inhalation, observe as the air naturally leaves your body, through your mouth, leaving you with the senses of divine fulfilment.

Slowly inhale and exhale for several breath cycles. Allow this process to focus your racing mind on the natural process of your breathing.

Let go of your thoughts. Witness your mind become more and more calm.

When you feel you are substantially focused, consciously bring the next inhalation in through your nose. As this inhalation is achieving completion, swallow. Thus, mixing the intake of this Chi filled breath with *Liquid Jade.*

As you now understand, many *Chi Kung* techniques witness you consciously directing your breath to your *Dan Tien.* With *Lien Chi,* however, you allow the breath to permeate your entire being. From this, you provide all elements of your being with positive Chi energy.

As was the case with *Pi Chi,* as you hold the *Lien Chi* breath in your body, count your heartbeats. Do not hold it until you are uncomfortable. Instead, release it when you feel it is necessary. As you do so, feel your entire environment becoming filled with positive Chi energy.

In the beginning, the practice of *Lien Chi* should be performed for a total of seven breath cycles. As you become more and more accustomed to it, you may proceed for as long as you feel comfortable with it and your mind remains focused. Many ancient Taoist monks are said to have performed this techniques as their sole source of meditation. Thus, it may take place for days, weeks, months, or even years in their mountain caves which they inhabited.

12 Gwar Chi

Gwar Chi means, *"Extending Chi."* This is an exercise where you begin to consciously release the Chi you have brought in and congregated inside of your body. This *Chi Kung* exercise is best performed directly after the *Lien Chi* exercise as your entire body is permeated with Chi.

This technique is commonly referred to as, *"Balloon Chi,"* as you mentally visualize a balloon in front of your body which you consciously fill with the Chi you are releasing.

Gwar Chi Exercise

Begin the *Gwar Chi* exercise in either a crossed legged stated posture or a standing position. Begin by taking a few natural breaths in through your nose, embracing its Chi power in your *Dan Tien* and then naturally exhaling via your mouth.

By this point in your *Chi Kung* advancement you undoubtedly are very consciously interactive with Chi. Thus, you can readily see it entering and empowering your being.

When you feel you are suitably prepared. Close your eyes and focus your next in-breath directly to your *Dan Tien.* Feel it expanding this region with golden light. Hold the breath for a total of seven heartbeats and then release it through your mouth.

Once it has been completely exhaled, experience its power for seven heartbeats and then bring in your next breath. As you do, extend your arms as if you are holding a large balloon. As the breath comes into your body, allow it to congregate in your *Dan Tien.* Hold it for seven heartbeats and then release it. As you do, see the golden Chi energy of this breath travel up your torso, out your arms, to the palms of your hands. Mentally visualize a balloon filling with the golden power of Chi which your body is unleashing from your hands. Mentally see the balloon fill to capacity.

Experience this for seven heartbeats and then take in your next breath, direct it to your *Dan Tien.* Release it and fill the balloon with golden Chi energy from your hands.

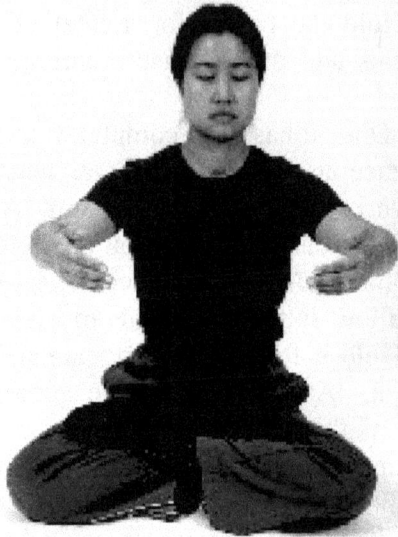

From this exercise you will initially learn to direct Chi to your hands to be used for any number of situations where you will need to unleash Chi energy for that part of your body. As you progress with this practice, you will begin to understand that the Chi you have taken in can be directed to any element of your body where it can be unleashed, as necessary.

13 Yun Chi

The Chinese term *Yun Chi* means, *"Transporting Chi."* This is the stage where you, as a *Chi Kung* practitioner, begin to not only be able to accurately focus Chi to specific regions of your body but to successfully extend it from your body, as well.

As you began to experience in the *Gwar Chi* exercise, you were able to redirect the Chi you brought into your body to a location outside of your physical being, (the imaginary balloon). In *Yun Chi* you take this understanding to the next level and actually begin to project Chi from your being.

Yun Chi: Exercise One

Move into a seated posture with your legs crossed. Close your eyes and begin to witness the natural process of your breathing. Focus your mind on that fact that Chi energy is coming into your body through your breath and filling you with unlimited universal energy.

After a few minutes of mental preparation, begin to consciously take in natural breaths and send them to your *Dan Tien.* Your breath comes in, it embraces your

Dan Tien with golden Chi light, it leaves but its power remains.

After approximately seven natural breath cycles, bring your arms up in front of your body with your fingers pointed upwards. Your palms should be facing each other, separated by approximately one foot. Become comfortable in this position as you continue to focus Chi energy into your *Dan Tien* with each in-breath.

When you feel comfortable, begin to send your exhalations out of your body via your hands. Mentally see Chi golden energy exiting your body from your fingers and your palms, forming a ball of golden Chi energy between your two hands.

With your new in-breath, breathe in more Chi energy, directed towards your Dan Tien. With your next exhalation, slowly bring your hands closer together as the breath leaves your body. You will immediately feel that there is a force emanating between your two hands.

Practice this technique for several breath cycles. Becoming increasingly aware of the power of Chi emanating from your hands.

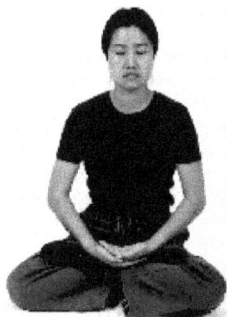

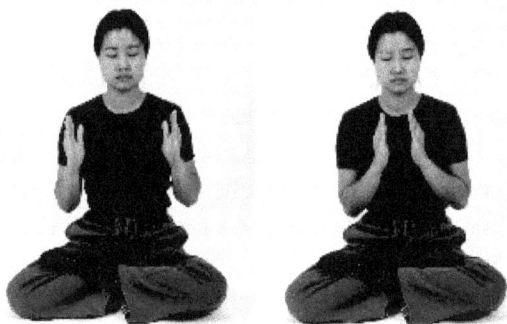

With this exercise you will quickly become aware of the fact that your hands are, in fact, projecting Chi energy. As you become more and more adept in your *Chi Kung* practices, you will be able to perform this exercise with little thought or preliminary focus. This is because of the fact, as you become more and more interactive with Chi, it will be continually emanating from your body. As your hands are direct tools for unleashing Chi energy, due to the fact that several Meridians culminate in them, you will be able to feel the power of Chi pulsating between them whenever your bring them together in this fashion.

Yun Chi: Exercise Two

This exercise is commonly referred to as, *"Pushing the Clouds," "An Yun Shou."* It can be performed from either a standing or seated posture.

Settle into your *Chi Kung* positioning, (either seated or standing), and watch your breath for a few moments as you become mentally focused. When you feel you are ready, close your eyes and bring your hands up to your chest level, with your palms facing forward. At the point you feel comfortable in this positioning, usually after several natural breath cycles, very consciously take in a slow Chi filled breath through your nose. See it entering your body in the form of golden light as it travels to your *Dan Tien,* illuminating it.

Begin to mentally visualize a white cloud directly in front of you. As you exhale your Chi filled breath, mentally witness it traveling up your torso, out your arms, and exiting your body via the palms of your hands.

As you breathe out, slowly extend your arms as this Chi filled breath exits via your palms. As your arms extend, see your internal energy pushing back on the cloud, causing it to move away from you.

Once you have completed your exhalation, leave your arms extending, pushing against the cloud, for a few moments. When it is time, breathe in another golden Chi filled breath, directed to your *Dan Tien*. As you do, slowly retract your arms to their original positioning as the cloud moves in closer to you. With inhalation completed, again, release it as you push the clouds away from you.

This technique can be used to push the clouds in whichever direction you feel most appropriate. It trains you to consciously direct Chi to your hands and to send it out via a very refined format.

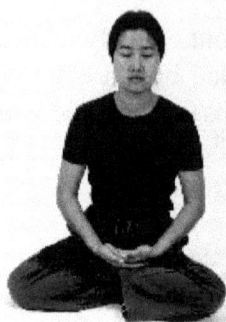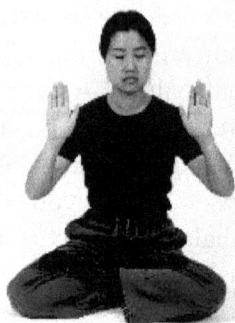

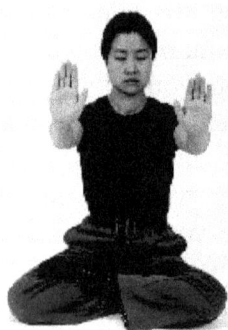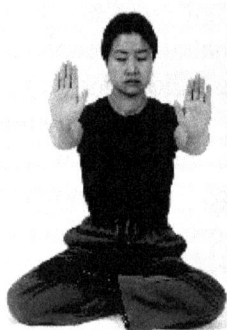

14 Chi and Physical Movement

Physical movement naturally stimulates the Chi in your body. From a physiological standpoint, it is commonly understood that the person who frequently exercises is the most physically and mentally healthy. The reasoning for this is twofold: from exercise, your heart beats with increased vigor. Not only does this stimulate this very vital organ but it also causes additional blood to pump through your veins, thereby nourishing and invigorating all aspects of your physical being. In addition, it has been scientifically proven that from physical movement your brain releases hormones. These hormones are known to create a more positive mental attitude.

The understanding of physical movement, in association with overall well-being, has been documented in China for centuries. It has long been known that movement naturally stimulates Chi that causes additional amounts of this universal energy to natural flow through your Meridians, thereby, causing your entire physical and spiritual being to enter into a state of enhanced universal balance and health.

Tai Chi Chaun

The Chinese exercises commonly known as, *Tai Chi Chuan,* are made up of exacting physical movements which are understood to cause Chi to be stimulated in the physical body.

Tai Chi Chaun, translated from the Chinese, literally means, *"Fist of the Supreme."* This physical science was developed during the fourteenth century in China. It evolved from the formalized movements of warfare, which monks and soldiers commonly practiced in relation to their various schools of martial arts. Therefore, *Tai Chi Chaun* is actually a form of the martial arts and was not initially developed as a means of precisely stimulating Chi energy.

From the late seventeenth century forward, however, this physical art form has evolved to the level where its techniques are employed in the realms of *Chi Kung.* This has occurred predominately by slowing down the offensive and defensive movements of *Tai Chi Chaun* to the degree where they have become more a form of movement meditation, than that of solely a means of defensive martial arts. None-the-less, though this is certainly not a negative aspect of the art, it must be understood that *Tai Chi Chaun* is still predominately considered an advanced form of self-defence. As such, Chi interactiveness is limited by the arts concentration on self-defense orientated movements.

Due to the indoctrination of many modern practitioners, they believe that martial arts and *Chi Kung* are, in fact, elementally the same. Historically, this is not the case. Though these two arts are now oftentimes intermingled, their origin and essence are quite different.

Formulated Chi Kung Movement

In order for you to gain a more precise understanding of how physical movement consciously stimulates Chi flow through your being, following are examples of prescribed movements which pick up where the *Yun Chi* exercise left off and cause Chi to come in, move through, and be directed out of your body, in association with physical movement. From these techniques you will learn how to cause Chi to actively enter your body and be redirected while you are consciously in a state of motion.

Chi Movement: Exercise One

Begin by standing with your feet apart, slightly wider than your shoulders. Rest your arms to your side, with your open palms facing your upper legs. Allow your fingers to extend in a relaxed fashion. Let them to be loosely separated.

Allow yourself a few moments to become comfortable in this positioning, as you begin to visualize Chi energy naturally entering your body through your nose with each in-breath and extending downwards to your *Dan Tien*.

Seven Heart Beats

During this exercise each of your inhalations, retentions, exhalations, and time between breaths will last for a period of seven heartbeats. This seven heart beat formulation was defined by ancient *Chi Kung* masters as the ideal time for the advancing student to meditatively bring their body and mind into harmony as they becomes acutely focused on the retention and transmission of Chi.

As in all cases of *Chi Kung,* if this seven heart beat time period is too long or you become uncomfortable during the process, breathe more frequently. If your are going to breath with a shorter duration, however, do so in a constant pattern in association with your heart beat; be it every seven beats, five beats, three beats, or two beats.

A natural occurrence of *Chi Kung* is that as you advance, you will be able to extend your breath cycle for more than a seven-heartbeat period, if desired. This is due to the fact that as Chi becomes more pervasive of your physical and spiritual being, you body becomes permeated with life giving Chi. Thus, breath is taken in much more conscious and, thereby, is used much more efficiently by your body.

Breathe and Count
Begin this *Chi Kung* process of heartbeat counting by consciously focusing your mind on the power of Chi. Breathe in slowly through your nose as you mentally witness your seven heartbeats. As you do so, consciously direct this in-breath to your *Dan Tien*. Once your inhalation is complete, hold it for a count of seven heartbeats, as the Chi energy radiates from this essential bodily location. Upon the seventh heat beat, release the breath through your nose as you witness seven beats. Then, experience your Chi filled breath emptiness for a count of seven.

Experience the Count
Before you begin the physical movements of this, or any *Chi Kung* exercise, allow yourself some time to become very accustomed to this meditative, heart beat counting process. For many individuals it takes a substantially amount of time to truly become meditatively focused to the degree where they can consciously experiencing their heartbeats, in association with breathing. For this reason, do not force

this process. If you do, the benefits of *Chi Kung* are lost.

It may take several days or longer for you to become accustomed to the initial level of this *Chi Kung* technique. But it is essential that you do so. There is no need to rush, simply allow yourself to naturally embrace with this process before you move further into its practice.

Begin to Move with Chi

At the point you have achieved the ability to naturally witness your heart beats, in association with your breath control techniques, move forward onto the physical aspects of this exercise. Begin, as a Chi filled breath comes into your body, via your nose, by slowly raising your arms. Bring them natural up in front of your body, directed by your shoulder muscles. Your palms should be allowed to turn to a downward facing position, parallel to the ground. Your wrists should not be held in a tight fashion. Instead, they should be allowed to bend slightly as no muscle pressure should be placed upon this region of your body. This initial inhalation and arm raising process should be achieved slowly, reaching its culmination with completion of your seventh heartbeat.

With the completion of your in-breath and your arms reaching shoulder level, enter into the period of Chi breath retention, leaving your arms in place as you observing your heart for seven natural beats. As you do so, feel Chi empowering your entire physical and ethereal being, as it congregates and emanates from your *Dan Tien*.

When this element of the exercise has been completed, slowly exhale, via your mouth, for seven heartbeats, as you lower your arms downwards in front of you. As your arms lower, see golden Chi emanating from your palms and impacting the Earth in front of you.

With the completion of the seventh heartbeat exhalation, naturally hold your palms in a downward facing position, as you embrace the emptiness of no breath coming into your being for seven heartbeats. See how you have now become interactive with Chi radiating between your body and the ground in front of you.

This exercise should be performed for a series of seven complete cycles. From this *Chi Kung* not only will you have allowed your body and mind to become meditatively focused but also you will have brought them into conscious harmony with your ethereal being. In addition, you will begin to become consciously interactive with that fact that you can cause Chi to be launched from a bodily part, direct it to a specific physical location, in this case the ground in front of you, and cause it to become naturally reflective.

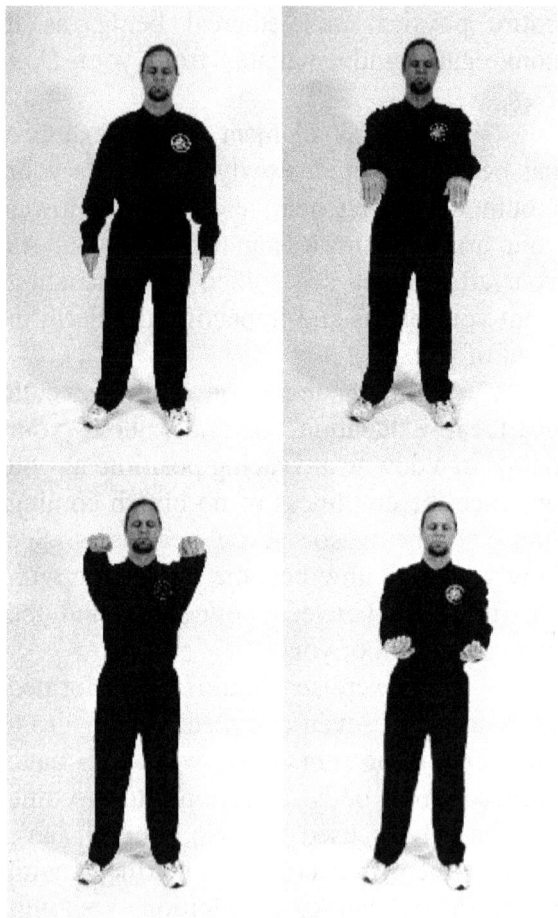

Energy Attracts Energy

As in all cases, energy attracts energy. This is especially true with Chi. Therefore, as you advance with this exercise, you will begin to see how the Chi directed from your palms, actually returns to your body, bringing with it additional power and invigoration.

Chi Movement: Exercise Two

This *Chi Kung* is performed in the same seven heart beat cycle as with *Chi Movement: Exercise One*. As with the case of the previous *Chi Kung* exercise, begin by standing with your feet naturally apart, slightly wider than your shoulders. Rest your arms to your side, with your open palms facing your legs. Allow your fingers to extend in a natural and relaxed fashion. Provide yourself a few moments to become meditatively comfortable in this positioning, as you become interactive with Chi by focusing on its power as you consciously bring it into your body via your breath.

When you feel that you have become interactive with Chi, begin by inhaling a slow seven heart beat breath through your nose and raising your arms from their resting position up in front of your body, with your palms facing towards the ground, *as your did in Chi Movement: Exercise One.* As you do, simultaneously move your legs into what is known as, *The Horse Stance.*

The Horse Stance

The Horse Stance is achieved by stepping to the side with your right leg, causing your feet to be located several inches outside of your should width. As soon as your step is completed, you slowly lower your body down by bending your knees. This causes your body to enter into a very firm positioning.

As you enter your *Horse Stance,* your arms continue to progress upwards. Instead of halting your movement at shoulder level, allows your hands to flip back, as your elbows arch, until your palms are facing towards the sky. This entire physical movement should be orchestrated to culminate with the completion of your seventh heartbeat in association with you inhalation.

Leave your arms in place, as hold your Chi filled breath for seven heartbeats – mentally encountering the power of Chi emanating in your *Dan Tien* and traveling up your torso and out your arms.

At the point your seven heart beat cycle has taken place, slowly exhale through your mouth as your powerfully push your arms up to the sky – tightening all of the muscles in your arms, upper body, and legs. As you do, mentally witness powerful golden Chi energy emanating from your palms, pushing a pure white cloud above your head. This technique is named, *"Lifting the Sky."*

Dynamic Tension

Commonly known as, *"Dynamic Tension,"* this physical muscle tightening, used in association with Chi breath control causes your Meridians to become invigorated with Chi. Thus, not only do your develop physical muscle strength but internal energy, as well.

When your exhalation and seven heartbeats have been completed, slowly allow your arms to return to their resting position at your side, as a period of seven heartbeats elapses.

See Page 148

You will notice that your heartbeat has increased as you have performed this segment of the exercise. From a physiological standpoint, this has naturally occurred due to the fact that you have exerted physical energy, causing your cardio vascular system to be stimulated. From a *Chi Kung* perspective, this has occurred due to the fact that you have stimulated the Chi flow along your Meridians. Thus, both the physical and ethereal element of your being has become nourished.

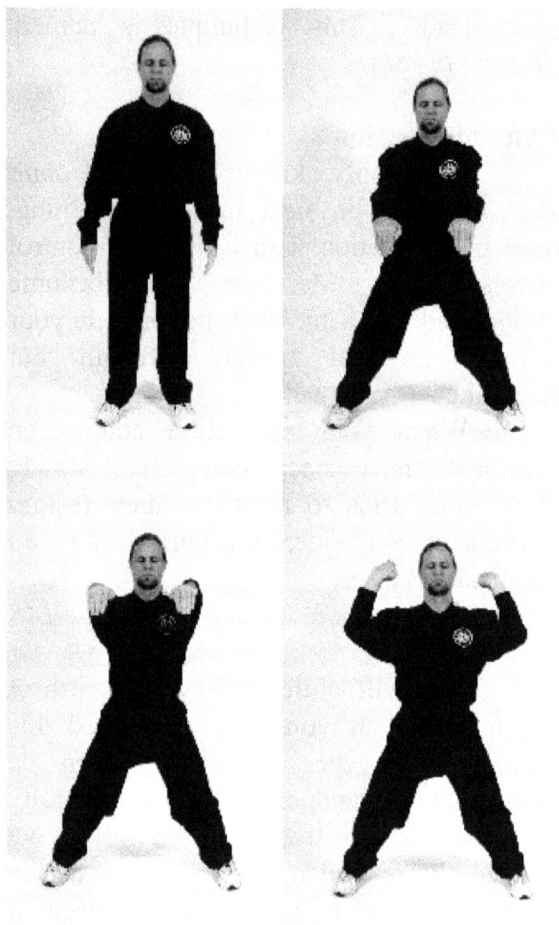

Allow your hands are at rest to your side, experience Chi filled emptiness for seven heartbeats. Then, perform this exercise again for a total of seven repetitions.

Chi Movement: Exercise Three

Begin as you did with the previous two exercises begin by standing with your feet apart, slightly wider than your shoulders, your arms naturally resting to your side. Always allow yourself several minutes to become consciously interactive with Chi before you proceed with the exercise.

This exercise also utilizes the seven heart beat *Chi Kung* formula. Therefore, upon the completion of your initial focalizing breaths, place your concentration upon your heart and begin to breath in association with seven beat.

When you have prepared yourself, with your next conscious inhalation of Chi breath via your nose, in a slow natural fashion, step forward with your right leg in a non-formal *Front Stance.*

The Front Stance

The Front Stance is accomplished by placing your right foot forward, approximately two feet in front of your left leg. Your rear leg remains straight, as your lead leg is allowed to lightly bend at knee level.

The Chi Hand

In association with this leg movement, raise your right arm until your palm is facing forward and your first finger is pointing directly upwards. Your other fingers should be allowed to bend slightly.

As the Large Intestine Meridian culminates in this finger, when you place your hand in this formation, it becomes a very powerful Chi defining tool that is commonly referred to as, *"The Chi Hand."*

This inhalation movement process should be coordinated to culminate with the completion of your seventh heartbeat. Once you have moved into this position, feel the Chi emanating from your *Dan Tien* as you body settles into this power filled positioning for seven natural heartbeats.

When the seventh beat has been experienced, exhale through your mouth as you extend your right arm with power and focus – mentally witnessing Chi traveling from your *Dan Tien,* out your arm, and being extended in front of your body from your right palm.

As you did with *Chi Movement: Exercise Two,* your arm, upper body, and leg muscles are tightened as your Chi empowered arm is extending. This movement should reach its completion as your seventh heartbeat occurs.

With the culmination of this phase of the exercise, slowly step forward with your left leg into a *Horse Stance,* as your arms come to a resting position. Embrace the Chi filled emptiness of a seven heart beat cycle. When this has reached its completion, move forward performing the same *Chi Kung* technique with your left arm.

This Chi orientated physical movement exercise can be performed up to seven times in order to focalize, direct, and empower you body with Chi.

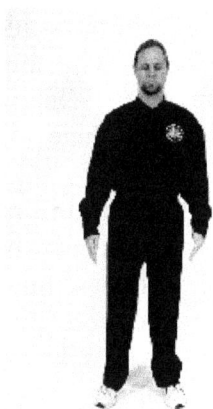

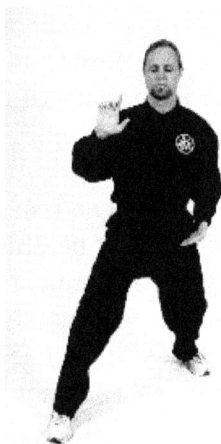

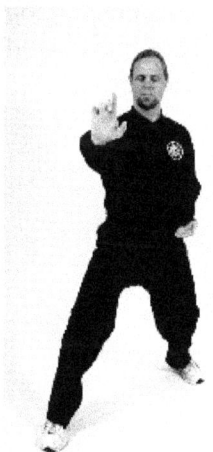

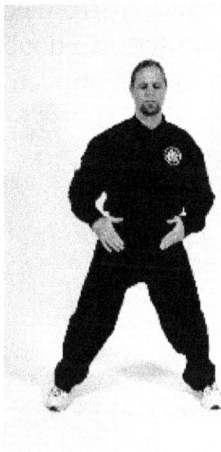

Movement and Chi

It must be ultimately understood that as you progress in *Chi Kung* and come to understand the interactive movement of universal energy in a more profound manner, you will realize that any and all physical movement actually stimulates your Chi. This is because of the fact that physical movement causes you to interact with the profound energies of this universe. Which, as detailed, are all in a constant state of vibration.

To this end, movement is movement. You should not be afraid to create your own patterns of movement which will cause you to become consciously interactive with Chi. Your move technique can be as simply as standing up and moving your arms slowly from side to side. Even from this simple movement, performed with a focus upon Chi, you will, no doubt, begin to understand interactive Chi movement consciousness.

15 Shou Kung

Shou Kung means, *"Long Life Technique."* This is the exercise which you should perform at the end of all of your *Chi Kung* sessions is order to not only focus this energy into your body but to additionally cause it to to remain in your *Dan Tien* in the form of *Nei Chi, "Inner Chi."*

Shou Gong Exercise

Enter into a standing posture. Close your eyes and experience the vitality you are experiencing due to the *Chi Kung* techniques you have performed. Feel the revitalizing energy permeating your entire being.

Begin to focus your mind on your *Dan Tien.* Place your hands loosely in front of it, with your fingers pointing towards one another, but not touching. Calmly bring in a breath through your nose. As you do, slowly bring your hands up to approximately your chest level. When it is time to naturally exhale, do so as your palms pivot over, facing the ground. As you breathe out via your mouth, slowly lower your hands to the region of your *Dan Tien.* With the exhalation complete, turn your hands over, palms facing upwards and perform this practice again.

This *Chi Kung* should be performed for approximately three to seven session or until you feel calm with your new Chi fully embraced by your entire physical and spiritual being.

16 Tsao Wong

Tsao Wong means, *"Sitting and Forgetting."* This term refers to the practice of formal seated meditation.

Tsao Wong is the final stage of *Chi Kung.* At this point of personal advancement, Chi flows through the body of the practitioner completely unhindered. Thus, the practitioner no longer is even concerned with its presence, as it is elementally embraced. With this level of Chi interaction, the focus is placed solely upon seated meditation in order to reach the state of *Wu, "Cosmic Nothingness."*

Meditation and You

You do not have to be at the point where you have experienced pure interactive cosmic consciousness with the universe to begin to meditate. In fact, meditation is one of the most beneficial actions you can perform in order to lead yourself into this sought after consciousness. This is because of the fact that through meditation you train your mind to become quiet to the degree where the advanced understandings of self-knowledge and universal communion may be embraced.

Wu

As discussed, *Wu,* or *"Cosmic Nothingness"* has been the sought after plateau of *Chi Kung* practitioners throughout history. *Wu* is an abstract concept to the average individual because of the fact that most people seek only to fulfill their momentary desires, as temporary as they may be. Thus, they never attempt to step back and embrace the, *action of inaction,* detailed in the *Tao Te Ching.*

Wu and Desire

The embracing of *Wu* initially witnesses you consciously letting go of your wants and desires. As it is understood that desires set you apart from enlightenment because they are all encompassing and are never ending.

How many times have you wanted something or someone with such intensity that you did everything in your power to obtain this desired passion? Once you received it, did the fulfillment of that desire answer all of your needs as you thought that it would? Or, did it simply move you forward onto new and different desires?

In virtually all cases, desire never provides you with any everlasting peace or contentment. Not only does the desire for something set you out of balance with peace but the obtaining of it does, as well. As desires never equal inner peace, the *Chi*

Kung practitioner consciously moves beyond this very low level of human consciousness and moves towards *Wu*.

Wu is consciously embraced but never desired. For centuries it has been understood that *Wu* is most readily encountered behind the veil of meditation.

Wu Shi

Wu Shi, is translated as, *"Five Periods."* This symbolized the stages the *Chi Kung* practitioner advances through until they obtain the level where *Wu* is experienced.

The five stages are:

1. The restless mind

2. The mind begins to calm

3. Internal balance and calmness are embraced.

4. The *Chi Kung* practitioner begins to be able to acutely focus and meditate.

5. The mind abides in stillness.

Tsao Wong Exercise

Meditation is a process of mental refinement that witnesses you sitting for a prescribed period of time each day and mentally focusing your mind upon a specific object. As breath is the delineating factor to the *Chi Kung* practitioner, breath should be the focus of your meditation.

Sit in *Lotus Posture* in the most peaceful environment you can find. Allow your hands to rest upon your lap, palms exposed, with your right hand lightly atop your left. Close your eyes.

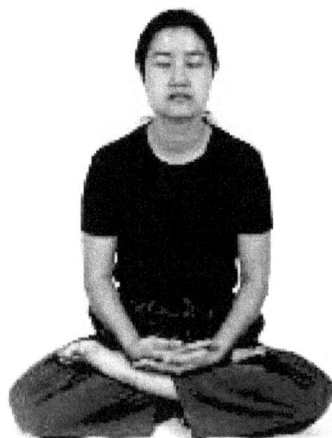

Begin by simply embracing the initial peacefulness you meet as you consciously sit down, close your eyes, and shut yourself off from the world. Do not attempt to do or think anything, just let yourself be at peace.

After a few moments of this initial practice begin to become consciously aware or your breath. Simply watch it entering your body, providing you with life and, then, naturally exiting your body. Do not attempt to control this process in any way. Simply witness it.

As meditation allows you time to be free from thinking, do not focus on any thoughts. Certainly, we are all trained to think all the time and have, in fact, become very accustomed to this process. But, let go of your thoughts. Each time you find yourself thinking about a situation that previously occurred or a desire you may have, let go of that thought and refocus your attention upon your incoming and your outgoing breath.

Many people become frustrated when they initially begin to meditate as their mind is constantly bombarded with thoughts. Do not let this bother you, it is natural, and in time will go away through meditative practice. Whenever a though comes to you, watch it fly away like a beautiful bird on the horizon and, again, refocus your attention upon your breathing.

To some they are very surprised that the process of meditation is based on such a simple premise – the witness of the incoming and the outgoing breath. But this is your key to life, why should you focus on anything else?

Watch your breath come in and witness it go out.

An appropriate time frame for meditation is half an hour in the morning and half an hour at night. In the early stages, however, do not force yourself to sit longer than you feel comfortable – ten of fifteen minutes is fine. After meditating for a time, this period will naturally extend.

Never force meditation, simply embrace the peace that it provides you.

Conclusion

As you progress with your understanding and conscious interaction with Chi you will come to realize that not only have you enhanced your own physical and mental conditioning but you will be empowered with high levels of Chi and have the ability to help other people. Some individuals become protective of these newly acquired skills and are reluctant to share this knowledge with others. From this type of possessive mental attitude, a person commonly throws their own body and mind out of alignment with the natural patterns of the universe. From this, the *Chi Kung* techniques which once helped them to gain newfound energy and cosmic understanding begin to cause them to encounter just the opposite and they begin to be plagued by the same Meridian blockages which they previously eliminated.

For this reason, as you progress further with the enhanced health and personal empowerment which is a by-product of *Chi Kung*, it is imperative that you use this newly acquired understanding to help others who have not yet been exposed to these ancient techniques. From this, you will not only enhance the physical, mental, and spiritual health of other human beings but you will add to the overall positive energy of this planet.

Glossary

Bodhidharma: India monk who traveled to China in 520 C.E. and became the Abbott of the Shaolin Monastery.

Buddhabhadra: (359-429) India Buddhist monk who traveled to China.

Chang Chueh: (114-184 C.E.) Founder of Tai Ping Tao, *"Way of Supreme Peace school."*

Chang Sheng Pus Su: Metaphysical immortality.

Chang Liang: (100 - 187 C.E.) Chinese Statesman.

Chang Tao Ling: (34 - 156 C.E.) Founder of *Five Pecks of Rice* school of Taoism.

Chen Jen: Pure Human Being.

Chi: Universal Energy.

Chi Kung: Method of consciously bringing Universal Energy into the human body.

Ching-i Tao: Way of Right Union School, 2nd Century C.E.

Ching Kung: Passive Chi Kung techniques.

Chi-po: The minister of Huang-ti.

Chuang Tsu: (369-286 B.C.E.) Chinese philosopher. Composer of *The Inner Chapters.*

Ch'u: Chinese State located in the Yangtze Valley.

Chu Lin Chi Hsien: *Seven Sages of the Bamboo Grove,* 3rd century C.E. Taoist sect.

Da Chang Jing: Large Intestine Meridian.

Dan Jing: Gall Bladder Meridian.

Dan Tien: Field of Elixir.

Fan Hu Zi: Reverse Breathing Chu Kung technique.

Fei Jing: Lung Meridian.

Fu Jin Hsiang: Meditative practice of absorbing Chi from the sun.

Fu Lu: Talismans.

Fu Shui: Holy water.

Gan Jing: Liver Meridian.

Gwar Chi: Extending Chi.

Huang-ti: The Yellow Emperor.

Huang Ti Nei Ching Su Wen: *The Yellow Emperor's Classic of Internal Medicine.*

Hsuan Hseuh: Secret Mystical Teachings. 3rd century C.E. sect of mystical Taoists.

Hsiao Pao Chen: 3rd century founder of Tai-i Tao.

I Ching: *Book of Changes.*

Jing: Meridians.

Jin Guang: Golden Light.

Kou Ch'ih: Chattering of the Teeth.

Kung Fu Tsu: Chinese Statesman and philosopher. More commonly known as Confucius.

Lao Tsu: Chinese philosopher. Composer of the *Tao Te Ching.*

Lien Chi: Melting Chi breath.

Lung Dong Bin: 7th century Chi Kung master.

Lun Yu: *The Analects of Confucius.*

Meng Tsu: (372 - 289 B.C.E.) Chinese philosopher, more commonly known as Mencius.

Nan Hua Chen Ching: *The Inner Chapters.*

Nei Chi: Internal Chi.

Nei Tan: Inner Cinnabar.

Pang Guang Jing: Bladder Meridian.

Pi Chi: Holding your Chi Breath.

Pi Jing: Spleen Meridian.

Sao Jian Jing: Triple Warmer Meridian.

Shen Hsien: 3rd century Taoist text detailing the method to immortality.

Shou Kung: Long Life Technique.

Shun Jing: Kidney Meridian.

Siddhartha Guatama: (563-483 B.C.E.) *The Buddha.*

Tai Chi Chaun: Fist of the Supreme.

Tai-i Chin Hua Tsung Chih: *The Golden Flower of the Supreme One.* 17th century text on Chi Kung.

Tai-i Tao: *Way of the Supreme Tao.* 13th century sect of Taoism.

Tai Ping Ching Ling Shu: *Book of Supreme Peace and Purity.*

Tai Ping Tao: *The Way of Supreme Peace* school of Taoism.

Tao: *The Way.*

Tao Hong Jing: (462-547 C.E.) Taoist healer.

Tao Te Ching: Book describing mystical Taoism.

Tao Yin: Stretching and Contracting the Body.

Tiao Chi: The Harmonizing of the Breath.

Tsao Wong: Sitting and Forgetting.

Tsou Yen: (350 - 270 B.C.E) Inventor of the Five Element understanding.

Tung Kung: Active style of Chi Kung.

Tun To: Chi Kung technique of consciously swallowing saliva.

Yen Chi: Swallowing the Chi Breath.

Yin and Yang: Shade and Light.

Yin Yang Chia: School of Yin and Yang.

Yu Chi: (124 - 197 C.E.) Taoist master.

Yun Chi: Transporting Chi.

Yu Chiang: Saliva

Yun Chi - Chi Chien: *The Cloud Book and Seven Strips of Bamboo.* 11th century text on Chi Kung.

Wai Chi: Outer Chi.

Wei Jing: Stomach Meridian.

Wang Ti: (226 - 249 C.E.) Taoist master.

Wu: Cosmic Nothingness.

Wu Hsing: Five Movers or Five Virtues.

Wu Shi: Five Periods.

Wu Tao Mi Tao: *Five Pecks of Rice* Taoism.

Wu Tsang: The Five Organs.

Wu Tsung: (814 - 850 C.E.) Chinese emperor.

Wu Wei: Non-Action.

Xian Chang Jing: Small Intestine Meridian.

Xin Bao Jing: Heart Constrictor Meridian.

Xin Jing: Heart Meridian.

Zhen Hu Zi: Normal Breathing Chi Kung technique.

Zim Chueng Shen: 7th century Chi Kung master.

Suggested Reading:

Campany , Robert Ford, Ge, Hong Shen Xian Zhuan. To Live As Long As Heaven and Earth: A Translation and Study of Ge Hong's Tradition of Divine Transcendence. Berkeley: University of California Press, 2002.

Davis, Edward L. Society and the Supernatural in Song China. Honolulu: University of Hawaii Press, 2001.

Ebrey, Patricia Buckley, Chinese Civilization: A Sourcebook. New York: Free Press, 1993.

Ebrey, Patricia Buckley. The Cambridge Illustrated History of China. Cambridge: Cambridge University Press, 1999.

Fisher-Schreiber, Ingrid, Ed., O'Neal, David, Ed., Wunsche, Werner, Trans. The Shambhala Dictionary of Taoism. Boston: Shambhala Publications, 1996.

Gernet, Jacques. A History of Chinese Civilization. Cambridge: Cambridge University Press, 1985.

Huang, Xiankuan. Chinese Qigong Acupressure Therapy: A Traditional Healing Technology for the Modern World. Bejing: Foreign Language Press, 2000.

Hymes, Robert. Way and Byway: Taoism, Local Religion, and Models of Divinity in Sung and Modern China. Berkeley: University of California Press, 2002.

Kohn, Livia, Roth Harold D., Ed. Daoist Identity. Honolulu: University of Hawaii Press, 2002.

Paludan, Ann, Wilkinson, Toby. Chronicle of the Chinese Emperors: The Reign-By-Reign Record of the Rulers of Imperial China. London: Thames & Hudson, 1998.

Pas, Julian F., Man Kam Leung. Historical Dictionary of Taoism. Landham: Scarecrow Press, 1998.

Pines, Yuri. Foundations of Confucian Thought: Intellectual Life in the Chunqiu Period, 722-453 B.C.E. Honolulu: University of Hawaii Press, 2001.

Roberts, J.A.G. A Concise History of China. Cambridge: Harvard University Press, 1999.

Sharf, Robert H. Coming to Terms with Chinese Buddhism: A Reading of the Treasure Store Treatis. Honolulu: University of Hawaii Press, 2001.

Shou-Yu Liang, Wu ,Wen-Ching. Qigong Empowerment: A Guide to Medical, Taoist, Buddhist, Wushu Energy Cultivation. East Providence: Way of the Dragon, 1996.

Strickmann, Michel, Faure, Bernard, Ed. Chinese Magical Medicine. Stanford: Stanford University Press, 2002.

Tzu, Shui-Ch'Ing, Ed., Cultivating Stillness: A Taoist Manual for Transforming Body and Mind. Boston: Shambhala Publications, 1992.

Wong, Eva, Trans. Harmonizing Yin & Yang. Boston: Shambhala Publications, 1997.

Wong, Eva. Teachings of the Tao: Readings from the Taoist Spiritual Tradition. Boston: Shambhala Publications, 1997.

Wong, Eva, Trans. The Shambhala Guide to Taoism. Boston: Shambhala Publications, 1997.

Wong, Eva, Trans. The Tao of Health, Longevity, and Immortality: The Teachings of Immortals Chung and Lu. Boston: Shambhala Publications, 1997.

Yang Jwing-Ming. The Root of Chinese Qigong: Secrets for Health, Longevity & Enlightenment. Boston: YMAA Publications, YMAA Publications.

www.ingramcontent.com/pod-product-compliance
Lightning Source LLC
Chambersburg PA
CBHW060432090426
42733CB00011B/2248